Ne

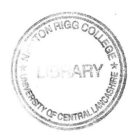

A GUIDE TO
CYCLING
INJURIES
PREVENTION & TREATMENT

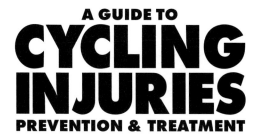

A GUIDE TO
CYCLING INJURIES
PREVENTION & TREATMENT

Dr Domhnall MacAuley

SBL

© 1995 Domnhall MacAuley MD MRCGP MFPHMI DPH DRCOG Dip Sp Med DSMSA

This edition first published by
Springfield Books, Norman Road,
Denby Dale, Huddersfield HD8 8TH

First Edition 1995

British Library Cataloguing in Publication Data
A catalogue record for this book is available from the British Library

ISBN 1 85688 048 6

Acknowledgements
The author and publishers would like to thank Mark Wohlwender
for the cover photograph

Designed and illustrated by Ian Chatterton

Printed and bound in Hong Kong by Colorcraft

To Skipper and First Mate!

CONTENTS

Introduction   8

1 The crash   10   Bunch riding   11
                                 Helmets   12
                                 Gravel rash   13

2 Treatment of   Physiotherapy   16
  minor injuries   Spine and neck injuries   17
  and conditions   15   Head injuries   17

3 The body   19   Injuries to the upper limbs 19
                                 Injuries to the lower limbs 25
                                 Injuries to the trunk   38
                                 Groin injuries   41

4 The muscles   44   Physiology   46
                                 Muscle fibre type   50

5 Stretching exercises 54

6 Hygiene   59

7 Training   62   How does training work?   62
                                 Overtraining   67

8 Weight training   72

9 Racing   78   Pre-race training   78
                                 Equipment   79
                                 Before the race   79
                                 Stage racing   80
                                 Diet   80
                                 Illness and Injury   82

10 Training your mind	**84**	Training period	84
		The race	85
		Psychological preparation	86
11 Winter training	**87**	Types of training	87
		Winter clothing	94
12 Your intake	**96**	Nutrition	96
		Fluid	100
		Alcohol	100
13 Drugs	**106**	Stimulants	106
		Narcotic analgesics	107
		Anabolic steroids	107
		Beta blockers	108
		Diuretics	108
		Peptide hormones	108
		Blood doping	109
		Local anaesthetic and steroid injections	109
		Other manipulative procedures	109
14 Ailments and minor handicaps	**111**		
15 Young cyclists	**121**	Overuse injuries	121
		Heat loss	122
		Psychological problems	122
		The heart	122
		Training and racing	122
Index	**124**		

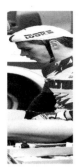

INTRODUCTION

Cycling is a sport that offers everyone an opportunity to participate, male and female, young and old, all shapes and sizes, regardless of physiology. Cyclists may race, tour or simply exercise to keep fit. For those wishing to race the sport offers opportunities to compete on the track, on the road, in sprints and in the ultimate long-distance endurance events. From the young and trendy enthusiasts with bronzed, oiled legs and the very latest in cool shades, to the older, overweight and slightly embarrassed first timers who simply wish to exercise for their health, cyclists all have in common, a love of the open road, a following wind, the sun on their back, and the ensuing sense of well being.

Cycling offers you the opportunity to enjoy a relatively safe sport, improving your health with little of the trauma associated with many other sports. The muscle action involves mainly the lower limb with sustained activity of muscle groups across three main joints, the hip, knee and ankle. In anatomy and physiology cycling draws comparison with running and long-distance rowing. Many believe that the main activity in cycling is the push on the pedals, however, contrary to popular understanding cycling is not a contraction and thrust movement but a rotation demanding the action of muscles in co-ordinated sequence throughout the pedal revolution.

Injury is uncommon as cycling is non-weight bearing and thus escapes the common repetitive trauma injuries of other endurance sports. Most typical running injuries are due to the long periods spent pounding the pavements, but in cycling the action is smooth and non jarring making injuries less likely, however they can occur when considerably longer periods are spent training and racing than in most other sports. Then there are patterns of overuse injury peculiar to cycling.

The intensity and duration of cycle training and racing means that nutrition is very important. For enthusiasts, who spend long periods training and racing this usually means taking great care with food intake. For many older cyclists burning those excess calories in the saddle is an ideal way to lose weight. At the other end of the nutritional spectrum the nature of extreme endurance events such as the Tours of France, Italy, and Spain demonstrate how cycling can be a considerable challenge to nutritionists. Indeed the dietary requirements of sustained periods of relatively intense physical activity even in domestic events have been dealt with by the athletes empirically: their caloric input defies many of the concepts of nutritional theory!

In spite of its safety record, accidents and injuries do happen. The most common are included in this book, together with prevention – where possible – and treatment based on medical training, common sense and hard-earned experience. Many of the injuries I see could have have been prevented with a bit more planning and care.

Within each section you will find a mixture of advice, from equipment to first aid, from self-help remedies to explanations of hospital treatments. The idea is to get you on your bike and to get the best from your cycling – as painlessly as possible!

CHAPTER 1

THE CRASH

There is little point in discussing the minutiae of physiological preparation and treatment of overuse injuries if we neglect one of the most common and preventable forms of injury: the crash. Perhaps in a book that concentrates on body maintenance a section on cycle maintenance is unexpected. However, there are certain basic aspects of cycle maintenance that are critical to the safety of both you and other riders in the race bunch.

Your bike should be safe, reliable and well maintained. It may seem obvious that wheels should be of good quality, well built and reliable. The rims and spokes should be of the necessary quality to withstand the rigours of a race, the pot holes, ramps and bumps on the road. Tyres should be of good quality with good tread and not worn. Tubular tyres, if used must be of good quality, but probably most important of all they should be stuck down well either with rim cement or tub-tape.

Brakes should work. They should be well maintained with good quality brake blocks and cable. The cable must be well secured. The cyclist may need to pull very strongly on brake levers at a critical moment so both the cable and the brake mechanism should be of sufficient strength and quality to withstand a maximum grip contraction.

The bike frame and forks should be sound. Naturally you should inspect the frame regularly for cracks or signs of weakening due to rust. For carbon fibre and aluminium frames it may be necessary to check the joints in the frame to ensure they are still secure. Carbon fibre frames should not be cleaned with spirit solvent as that may weaken the adhesive.

Pedals and cranks should be well secured, toe straps should be of good quality leather, not worn or frayed. If you use clipless pedals the pedal and shoe plates should be adjusted properly.

Pre-race bike checks prior to the 'sign on' are often considered an irritating and unnecessary part of bicycle racing. However each of us should welcome a compulsory bike check. We should be confident that our own bikes are safe and reliable; and the bike check ensures that every other bike is equally safe. We have all witnessed crashes due to equipment failure, but the most irritating aspect is that these crashes are preventable. We may maintain our bikes for our own safety, but we must always be aware of the great danger posed to others when a crash could be caused through poorly maintained or inadequate equipment. There should be a group awareness of the necessity to maintain a high standard of equipment, such that we are quite prepared to point out to a fellow competitor if poor quality or maintenance of his or her equipment is putting us all at risk.

BUNCH RIDING

There is a certain code of conduct when riding in a group. A foolish or careless move by any rider can easily reduce the racing peloton to a tangled wreckage of bodies and bicycles scraping along the road at 30 miles an hour. We should not only take care in our own behaviour in the bunch, but also be prepared to point out to others when they put us at risk. Experienced riders, amateur and professionals, will often complain of the risks in riding with competitors less experienced than themselves. In general, the more experienced the rider the more aware he is of the risks and dangers of riding in a bunch where mistakes can mean injury. The behaviour of some riders is not poor etiquette but frankly dangerous. Overtaking on the wrong side of the white line on a blind corner, or dodging among the traffic puts us all at risk. We see riders slipstream passing cars and vans, mount footpaths or threaten pedestrians. We see riders ignore marshals, or block motorcycle marshals from getting through, forgetting that they keep us safe by regulating the traffic, signalling hazards, and alerting the race director to road and traffic conditions ahead.

Cycling etiquette is not simply manners for the sake of politeness. It is a critical matter of safety, prevention of crashes, injuries and fatalities. It is not important just for the image of our sport, but any serious injury or fatality is not only a tragedy for the individual and their family, but also undermines the whole *raison d'être* for our sport.

HELMETS

Competing with the most basic headgear and racing at about 25mph and 40 to 60mph at times downhill, cyclists are extremely vulnerable. Cycling helmets are compulsory in amateur cycling and in most professional events. However cyclists often wear the minimum to conform with regulations. The simple leather straplike banana helmet, for example, provides almost no protection. The heavier hard shell or covered polystyrene type are much more effective.

It is interesting to note the changes in attitude among cyclists towards helmets. Usually the fashions and trends are set by high profile professionals. In this case, despite attempts by the international commissaires to enforce the regulation stipulating that professionals should wear hard shell helmets, most professionals have refused and most are seen in the media inadequately protected. However, at the same time leisure cyclists have begun to wear proper head protection. In cycle touring and leisure events, hard shell helmets are almost uniformly worn, although optional. It is ironic that although hard shell helmets were compulsory in amateur racing and are still worn by most, it is not unusual to see competitors cycling to and from events on busy roads with their helmets draped over their handlebars.

At the same time we must recognise that although a rider may be injured while racing, riders are just as vulnerable while training. It could be argued that protective headgear should be worn when riding the bike at all times: training, racing or simply going to the shops. Traditionalists may scoff, but it is interesting to note that helmets are compulsory under road traffic regulations in many other countries. Hard shell helmets have always been compulsory in triathlon and the rules are very firmly enforced.

Road traffic accident statistics and accident figures for children indicate that head injuries in leisure cycling are directly associated with non use of appropriate headgear. Although safety standards have been set there is great variation in the level of protection offered even among reputable manufacturers. It is important to ensure that the helmet conforms to the appropriate safety specification: ANSI or Snell.

One complaint voiced by cyclists is that helmets are too hot, especially when climbing during hot weather. There is very little evidence to support this. Most helmets are well ventilated with air ducts forming an integral part of the design. There may be some relevance to this complaint if climbing high mountains in the Alps or Pyrenees in mid summer but little justification in the UK or Ireland. Most new helmets have an integral hard shell but earlier designs had a polystyrene base under a nylon cover. It is essential to wear this cover over the shell but it is equally important that it allows easy air passage.

The most common complaint among cyclists is chronic neck strain, even though modern helmets are very light. Some riders suffer from an ache at the lower neck and across the shoulders. There is no easy answer other than to persist in wearing the helmet until your neck muscles adapt. Choosing between a stiff neck or a fractured skull isn't difficult – ALWAYS WEAR A HELMET.

GRAVEL RASH

The term gravel rash is a misnomer. It is used to describe the friction burns that occur when a cyclist falls, scrapes along the road and removes the top layer of skin from the hips, legs or arms. This top surface layer of skin may be torn off to varying degrees, sometimes down to the muscle. Gravel rash is **the** most common cycling injury. Gravel, oil, and other slippery agents on the road are a common cause of crashes and the drafting effect of cycling in a bunch is so great that, since cyclists ride in such close proximity, if one falls others inevitably fall too. Appropriate first aid facilities are an essential prerequisite of cycle race organisation.

With superficial friction burns there is merely loss of part of the superficial layer of skin. The skin itself remains intact but covers the damaged area with a liquid ooze or exudate. New skin grows from the lower layers underneath the exudate. With a deeper friction burn the entire layer of skin is lost and there is no skin underneath to repair the damage. New skin must grow from the edge of the wound and healing is much slower. When this new skin has formed being scar tissue, which is at first more rigid and more easily torn, it is not as supple and elastic as the original skin. Eventually this scar tissue recovers to be just as strong and supple as normal skin. Crashes are such a common occurrence in cycling that many professionals have large areas of scar tissue on their hips from recurrent injuries, an unfortunate part of the life of a professional cyclist.

When the integrity of your skin is damaged its protective layer is removed and the wound may be contaminated by pieces of gravel, glass, hay, cow dung, and other detritus from the road. If you fall and suffer gravel rash these contaminants must be removed to avoid infection of the wound. The wound must be cleaned as soon as possible. If sterile water and appropriate dressing packs are not available, and this is likely unless it is an international race where a doctor is available, then it is appropriate to clean the wound with copious quantities of tap water. Many cyclists keep a sponge in their kit bag for cleaning themselves. If you have a clean sponge then it may be used to wash out the wound, but never, never use a sponge to clean your own wound that has already been used by someone else. At times, with a severe gravel burn, a sponge is not sufficient to clean the pieces of gravel from a wound. In this case a toothbrush or nail-brush may be required. A doctor will inject local anaesthetic, to enable the wound to be cleaned more effectively. The traditional cycling hard man grits his teeth!

In order to minimise injury, cyclists often wear two layers of clothing, so when striking the road the two layers may slide over each other rather than abrade the skin. Racing cyclists shave their legs. One possible advantage is that this prevents leg hairs sticking to the serous exudate in the wound following a friction burn!

The next time you are planning your ride, see if you have room in your kit bag for a small sponge, a little bottle of sterile water, along with sticking plasters and a tube of antiseptic.

CHAPTER 2

TREATMENT OF MINOR INJURIES AND CONDITIONS

C ycling is relatively injury free. Unlike contact or collision sports such as rugby, soccer or Gaelic games, you the cyclist are unlikely to finish a race battered and bruised. However, you may injure yourself while out running, in the gym, or in a crash.

There are some basic principles in treating minor injuries to help recovery and ensure early return to sport. The principles of the treatment of common strains and sprains are: Rest, Ice, Compression and Elevation – **R I C E**. These guidelines are relevant for minor injuries only, and you should, of course seek medical advice if you are in any doubt.

- **ICE:** cools the skin and underlying tissue. This reduces swelling, helps prevent bruising, and has some pain relieving effect. Use whatever is available: ice cubes in a bag, a bag of frozen peas, proprietary iced strapping (bought in tins from sports shops) and pads, or simple ice application for two to three minutes. To ensure that the skin is not burned, the ice should be wrapped in a damp towel to avoid direct contact between the ice and skin. Ice application should be repeated every two to three minutes for approximately 20 mins.

- **COMPRESSION:** pressure from a bandage on the injured area helps prevent excessive swelling. The injured limb should be strapped in a compression bandage ensuring that compression is not so tight that it inhibits blood supply. A crêpe bandage or elasticated support such as a tubigrip may be sufficient.

- **ELEVATION:** raising the injured part can help reduce swelling. The injured limb should be held up, ideally above waist height. After injury there is oedema or swelling caused by fluid gathering around the injured part. Elevation reduces swelling by preventing accumulation of fluid in a dependent limb thus spreading the fluid. One important practical point is that following injury, you should not head off to the bar and stand for hours imbibing anaesthetic before treatment! A sprained ankle will only become more swollen, immobile and delay recovery. Ice, compression and elevation should be the immediate treatment, and early treatment means early recovery.

- **REST!** Rest is relative. An injury that needs rest means rest of the injured part but not total inactivity. Injury to a leg may keep you from cycling or running but should not prevent swimming or upper body circuits or weight training. You can swim or even run in the pool wearing a flotation jacket. The primary aim after any injury is rapid return to activity. Your return to cycling after injury may be much earlier than other sports due to the very nature of your sport.

Early mobilisation is an important principle. For example, after an ankle sprain sustained during winter training a typical programme to ensure rapid return to sport would consist of walking, followed by gentle jogging in straight lines. Then try running in straight lines with walking the turns, gentle jogging the turns, and finally running in large semi circles. When you can run and turn rapidly then you may return to training. The cyclist can often return to the bike much earlier than runners or other sportsmen, as the sport does not require great functional activity at the ankle joint. So after an ankle sprain, you can return to cycling within days.

PHYSIOTHERAPY

The process of recovery from injury does not end after first aid. Many injuries affect muscle function. Physiotherapy can offer various types of treatment including ultrasound, interferential and lasers. However, perhaps the most important aspect of physiotherapy is the hands-on practical approach. The physiotherapist is ideally suited to offer treatment and advice on rehabilitation and suitable retraining. Their training gives them particular understanding of the structure and function of muscle, optimum retraining and specific exercises in recovery. We are very lucky to have many very active and enthusiastic sports physiotherapists. However you should judge your physiotherapist not by the technology or sophisticated equipment available but by their knowledge and understanding of the needs of your sport.

MORE SERIOUS INJURIES

Serious injury does occur and we must always be on our guard. A sprain may be a fracture! Fractures must be dealt with at hospital and careful heed must be paid not to worsen the injury by careless management. The use of a splint will ensure maintenance of good position, least pain and adequate blood supply.

SPINE AND NECK INJURY

Spinal injuries can occur and the results of such injuries are devastating. Depending on the level and extent of the injury, partial or complete paralysis may occur. In a serious accident we must ensure that first aid treatment is appropriate to ensure no further damage.

Commissaires, officials and other racers must be especially aware of possible injury following a crash. An injured cyclist who complains of a neck or back injury must not be moved. An ambulance, which has the facilities to lift the patient with a scoop stretcher should be called. The race, if a circuit race must be stopped and if necessary abandoned to enable the injured to be taken to hospital. Complaints of back or neck pain must not be taken lightly. Any neck or back injury is potentially serious until proven otherwise.

HEAD INJURY

Concussion means brain damage! Even if only temporary, it is important not to underestimate its severity. Concussed cyclists should not remount and continue a race. They have sustained at least some temporary brain damage and are thus more likely to injure themselves or others, especially in a bunch. Concussion, however minor, may affect some mental function and in the close constant surging movements of the bunch, it is essential to be completely alert. Even a minor loss of judgement or co-ordination can mean disaster for many, so concussed riders must be withdrawn from a race.

The serious affects of head injury may not be immediately obvious so there are certain key rules to be observed. The effects of alcohol make it impossible to tell its effect from any possible brain damage or loss of coordination, so it is vital that you do not race and booze. Should you sustain a head injury, you should be accompanied home and relatives informed. If knocked out, or if suffering from headaches, double vision, or vomiting, you should attend hospital.

Advice following a head injury

You have just attended hospital and the doctor has found no evidence of serious head injury. From now on there should be a gradual improvement in your condition. For the next twenty four hours, however, you should not consume alcohol, drive a car or use any dangerous machinery and you should always have someone with you. Through the night you should be wakened every three hours.

If you, or whoever is with you, notices any of the following problems you should reattend hospital immediately:

- If you are difficult to rouse

- Vomiting (more than once)

- Severe or increasing headache, dizziness, drowsiness or double vision

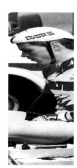

THE BODY

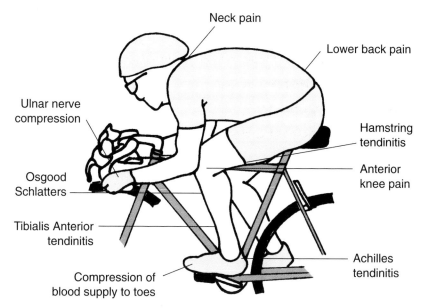

Neck pain

Lower back pain

Ulnar nerve compression

Hamstring tendinitis

Osgood Schlatters

Anterior knee pain

Tibialis Anterior tendinitis

Compression of blood supply to toes

Achilles tendinitis

INJURIES TO THE UPPER LIMB

There are three pressure areas in cycling: the hand on the handlebars, the foot on the pedals, and the perineum on the saddle. While knee injuries are the most common in cycling, injuries to the hand follow closely. These may be due to pressure of the hands on the bars, or due to trauma from falling off the bike.

The Hands

You can grip the handlebars in either of two ways:

- Hands on the tops. The wrist is in the neutral position, but hands are extended across the brakehoods with the web space between thumb and forefinger resting on the hood. This position is usually adopted when touring or during a more relaxed phase of racing.

● On the drops. During more important phases of racing when the handlebars must be gripped more tightly, the hands are positioned on the 'hooks' or drops ie the lower plane of the handlebars. The wrist is extended; the main pressure point being the base of the thumb and the flat of the hand.

Numbness and weakness of fingers

During a hard race or while riding over an uneven surface it is tempting to grip the handlebars very tightly. In gripping so tightly there may be considerable pressure on the front of the wrist and heel of the hand. This pressure may squeeze the front of the wrist and in particular the ulnar nerve. The ulner nerve gives sensation to part of the ring finger, the little finger and is the nerve to some of the muscles moving the fingers. The nerve divides into two branches at the heel of the hand and pressure may bruise either one or both branches.

Bruising occurs more often where the cyclist is a relative novice or where the race is over rough terrain and the athlete must grip tightly to control the bike. During difficult races over cobblestones professional cyclists commonly pad their handlebars. Padding not only reduces vibration from the cobble stones but also allows the cyclist to grip the handlebars without injuring the nerve. Pressure on the sensory branch can cause numbness of the little finger and the outer half of the ring finger. The numbness caused often eases some hours after the cycle ride and it is best not to return to cycling until this numbness has resolved, lest permanent damage result.

Pressure on the other branch of the nerve may cause temporary paralysis of some of the muscles of the hand. This branch is called the motor branch. The motor branch supplies the muscles that keep the fingers together. It may be be tested by trying to hold a sheet of paper between the fingers with the fingers straight.

Trauma to the hand

When falling off a bike, it is a natural reaction to put out your hands to break the fall. However the palms of the hand are easily injured during a crash by friction against the road surface. These injuries can be very severe, tearing the skin and deeper structures. Not only are such injuries slow to heal but the healing process itself can severely disable the rider. With a serious abrasion on the palm the skin heals with scar tissue. This scar tissue is not as supple and stretchy as normal skin. The scar tissue tightens up and leaves the injured cyclist with tight immobile hands and fingers. While skin on other areas of the body may heal with scar tissue, mobility of the hand is most important in all trades and professions, and the contractures resulting from healing hand injuries may be very disabling. New scarred skin may grow tight and thick and the hand will be less able to carry out fine detailed movements. Palm injuries healing with scar tissue and deformity may need plastic surgery at a later date.

You can protect yourself against this injury by wearing gloves. All racing cyclists should be encouraged to wear proper cycling mitts with a reinforced leather palm. The leather palm of the glove or track mitt will offer some protection and help prevent loss of the skin surface. Occasionally during a stage race, the leading rider and his team ride without track mitts so the numbers of opposing riders who are a threat on the general classification may be written on the backs of their hands. However they should be aware of the appalling problems of severe abrasion injuries to the hands.

Bone injuries

Falling can cause fractures to any bone of the upper limb from the tip of the finger to the shoulder depending on the nature of the fall.

The fingers

Most fractured fingers are relatively uncomplicated and while they cause pain, and inconvenience they are easily treated and usually heal well. The rider who suspects a finger is broken after a fall should seek hospital advice and confirmation by x-ray. Most bones should be splinted to improve healing and splinting of a finger is usually relatively easy where one finger is strapped to its neighbour. This is good news if you wish to return to training and racing as soon as possible. When the pain has eased, and providing you can grip the brakes and handlebars, you may return to training. A more complicated finger fracture may require a special splint which immobilises the finger more effectively meaning you will not be able to cycle on the road. Training may continue on the turbo trainer.

Injuries to the thumb are more serious. The thumb is used in almost every movement requiring manual dexterity and is necessary for grip at all times. Many thumb injuries require splinting or even surgery. Treat thumb injuries with respect.

The Wrist

Wrist fractures should be seen at hospital as even apparently minor breaks may need medical intervention, plaster cast and close follow up. The bones of the forearm are known as the radius and ulna. Fractures of these may need to be manipulated and plaster cast. It may often be possible to resume training on a turbo trainer fairly soon after treatment.

Fractures of the small bones that make up the wrist may or may not need close medical management. However, they all need to be assessed by x-ray. One of the more common and important wrist fractures is to the scaphoid. The scaphoid is a small and apparently insignificant bone which is situated at the junction of the wrist and the base of the thumb. However, injury to the scaphoid may give long term problems because it has a poor blood supply. Occasionally after a fracture, part of this bone may not heal causing later problems with pain and subsequent arthritis. Unfortunately this injury happens most often when falling with the hand outstretched, exactly the way most cyclists fall.

It is important to know how to identify this problem. If you cock your thumb back you may see two tendons standing out on the back of your wrist on the same side as the thumb. Between these two tendons is a dimple known as the 'anatomical snuffbox'. If after a fall off the bike it is painful to press in between these two tendons then seek help. This fracture may not show up immediately on an x-ray but needs to be put in plaster just the same. The doctor will usually arrange a further x-ray three weeks later to confirm the fracture. The plaster cast for this seemingly minor injury covers the entire wrist and thumb and making it impossible to grip the handlebars.

Fractures of the elbow require urgent medical assistance at a hospital. There are important nerves and blood vessels very close to the elbow joint and it is easy to damage these structures with a fracture. It is important to treat elbow fractures with respect. The cyclist who fractures an elbow may spend some time in hospital, may require surgery, and will most probably miss the entire cycling season.

The upper arm and shoulder

Fractures of the bone of the upper arm known as the humerus will require hospital assessment, but is usually treated with a form of sling. Return to the bike may be relatively early. Dislocation of the shoulder is unusual in cycling and is much more likely to occur in football or rugby. If it occurs the cyclist may be back training and racing in three weeks with good physiotherapy.

Fracture of the collar-bone or clavicle

This is perhaps the most common and best-known fracture to cyclists. Many famous international figures in professional cycling have had their season disrupted due to this injury, the most notable being the retirement of Sean Kelly from the Tour de France in 1989 and again the very same injury in the Spring of 1991. Rolf Sørensen crashed and fractured his collarbone while leading the Tour de France in 1991.

The clavicle, better known as the collar-bone, is a relatively unimportant bone whose main purpose is to keep your shoulders apart! You may feel the contours of the bone just under the skin crossing between the neck and shoulder. It keeps the shoulder joint away from the trunk so we may lift and carry.

When falling off the bike you usually put out the arm automatically to break the fall. Remember that when falling off a bike at 25mph the shoulder falls through about five feet and there is considerable momentum. It's easy to appreciate the considerable pressure being driven up the arm pushing the shoulder against the bony structure of the clavicle. This type of fall occurs in other sports but with much less force. For example: in rugby, especially in rugby league, shoulder sprains are common but the increased forces associated with cycling falls make fractures more common. As with any fractured bone it is rather painful. In most cases you would find it too painful to move the shoulder, let alone get back on the bike.

It is a reflection on the remarkable strength and courage of the man that on each occasion when Sean Kelly broke his collar-bone he remounted. On the first occasion during the Tour de France he was unable to continue, but in 1991 he remounted and completed the stage before withdrawing from the race. In most cases the cyclist will be taken to hospital for x-ray confirmation of the break.

What next?

As with any broken bone it is important to ensure that both ends of the bone meet for proper healing. In most cases this requires an anaesthetic while the doctor manipulates or operates on the bone to bring the ends together, but it is usually not necessary for collar-bone fractures.

With most other fractures the bone is immobilised in a plaster cast or splint so the ends remain together for recovery and to ensure there is no load on the healing bone. Once again, due to its relatively unimportant structural role and its small load, it is not essential to completely immobilise the collar-bone for recovery. It would be rather difficult to splint or put plaster of Paris on a collar-bone!

The usual treatment, after x-ray diagnosis, is to wear a sling and take pain relief. The bone does not need to be 'reduced' or put back in place. This fracture is simply left to heal on its own. Very often the two broken ends of the bone are not exactly in their natural position and the bone heals with a 'step'. Many athletes who have had a fractured collar-bone have a a bony lump or step along the contour of the clavicle.

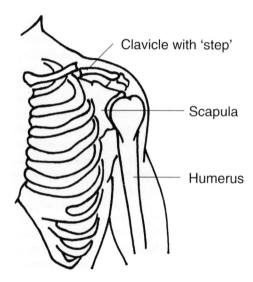

Clavicle with 'step'

Scapula

Humerus

Recovery

Recovery of most simple bone breaks in less important bones is about six weeks, as for example a broken wrist. The fractured collar-bone takes approximately the same time. However this does not mean that you cannot do any training. In a sense we are lucky, because although the fractured collar-bone is a relatively common injury in cycling, you may usually return to your bike earlier than to other sports.

For two weeks after a fracture, while the ends of the bone are just beginning to knit, the shoulder will be too painful to do much movement. After about two weeks the bone will have some stability, as the break heals initially with fibrous tissue and gristle. Although the gristle is not nearly as strong as bone you may return to the turbo trainer and use your legs without upper body movement.

As healing progresses, the shoulder will become more stable, less painful, and you may be able to train on your own bike on the road. Initially you should stay on flat roads with a good surface. Any rough surface or uneven terrain will cause jarring transmitted through the handlebars and cause collar-bone pain. In four to six weeks you should be able to return to normal cycling on the road, climbing, sprinting etc. The collar-bone, although quite well healed, is still relatively weak, and would be more susceptible to further injury should you fall.

Sean Kelly returned to racing five weeks after his collar-bone fracture in 1991. Rolf Sørensen took part in the 1991 Wincanton classic just three weeks after his fractured clavicle. Eight weeks would probably be a more realistic target for most of us. Mountain bikers may be advised to wait three months before returning to hard racing, as awkward falls are an integral part of the sport!

The collar-bone is a relatively unimportant bone. However due to the nature of cycling accidents, and our natural response in protecting ourselves, the fractured collar-bone has become one of the classic cycling injuries. It is always a disappointment when it occurs, usually in the middle of the racing season, but in terms of recovery and rehabilitation we are relatively lucky in that we can return to our sport relatively quickly. It can be painful, and who will forget the combination of pain and disappointment etched on the faces of Sean Kelly and Rolf Sørensen as we witnessed their respective withdrawals from Le Tour on worldwide television.

INJURIES TO THE LOWER LIMBS
Knee pain
Knee pain is almost an occupational hazard of cycling and overuse injuries of the knee are the most common of all cycling injuries. We can all identify with the many folk heroes of cycling who have suffered knee pain, often for long periods, threatening or even ending their career. Reading of the trials and tribulations of the top professionals often reveals that one of the most common injuries is the painful knee. Even our own friends and clubmates are not immune and many a conversation on the club run has centred on the cause, prevention and treatment.

Cycling at 100 rpm for four or five hours puts enormous stress on the knee. For some, knee pain is inevitable, but there is much we can do to try to prevent it.

The most common problem is pain behind the kneecap, sometimes felt just behind the inside edge, described as anterior knee pain. It used to be known as chondromalacia patella and this term is still used although it's not strictly correct. The kneecap slides up and down a groove on the thigh bone when the quadriceps muscle is contracted. The passage of the kneecap up and down within this groove depends on symmetrical pressures drawing on the kneecap. There are thus two mechanisms for development of knee pain: it may be due to a tracking or a loading problem.

● Excess load

If we think of the kneecap as a pulley for the thigh muscles as they cross the knee then we can understand how, if there is excess stress on the knee from excess load, the kneecap will be forced excessively against the leg bone. Healthy muscle can exert a force of 42 pounds per square inch and the quadriceps is a most powerful muscle exerting a force up to 700 pounds. The secret to prevention of excess load is cadence. Cycling at a higher pedal rate in a lower gear ensures that the bike travels at the same speed but with less pressure on the kneecap with each pedal stroke.

● Abnormal tracking

If in addition, the forces on the knee tend to draw the kneecap out of the groove then this will cause abnormal friction forces on the reverse side of the kneecap. Prevention of knee pain depends therefore not only on reducing loading on the knee but also in preventing alignment problems.

Training load

Knee pain may arise during the season for no apparent reason. The cyclist may simply note the onset of this nagging pain and be unable to relate it to any specific cause. However, careful analysis may reveal a precipitating factor:

● Sudden increase in mileage at the beginning of a season may be too much too soon.

● Competing in a major tour may demand very high mileage at high speed on successive days with a lot of climbing.

- Sometimes following a period off the bike due to illness or holidays you may try to compensate by increasing training mileage more than in preceding weeks at a time when gradual increase in training load would be more appropriate.

You should therefore avoid sudden increases in intensity or duration of training.

Cycling position

Saddle height

Cyclists should also avoid dramatic changes in their position on the bike, especially with a new frame or changing from training to a racing bike. The height of the seat is important at the onset of knee pain and you should check if you have made any recent adjustments in the height of your seat. Seat height adjustments should be made gradually. A good rule of thumb is to adjust seat height not more than one centimetre per week. It is important that the seat is not too high. Although the biomechanical principles seem unclear, there is no doubt that knee pain is more common with a saddle that's too high.

Many coaching books demonstrate the appropriate saddle height and how to achieve this.

Crankshafts

Cyclists may fit longer crankshafts in the belief that this will improve efficiency and power generation. Although of theoretical benefit, the alteration in length of crankshaft while giving greater torque means greater force to be applied by the legs with each stroke and lower cadence. Longer cranks put greater stress on the joint, more stress with each pedal stroke, and more likelihood of knee pain.

Pedals

The type of pedal used may have significant influence on the development of knee pain. Clipless pedals have been a recent revolutionary innovation; while they have been of great benefit to many cyclists, they have been associated with injury in others. Foot posture alters naturally throughout the pedal revolution. With clipless pedals there is less freedom of movement. The foot alters its position naturally and imperceptibly throughout the pedal stroke. In clipless pedals the foot is much more restricted and the body must compensate for this rigidity by rotatory movement further up the leg, in particular at the knee. This may precipitate maltracking already due to the rigid position of the foot during the pedal revolution.

Cleat pedals are manufactured for the anatomically perfect but we are all different and although some may have symmetrical feet and legs most of us are not biomechanically identical. Clipless pedals will emphasise any anatomical anomaly or biomechanical misalignment. If you have any tendency to knee pain then perhaps these pedals are not suitable. Manufacturers are aware of this shortcoming and have attempted to overcome the problem by increasing the amount of movement or play in the pedals. However at present this movement is only in a lateral plane whereas natural foot movements occur in all directions.

Climbing

Increase in climbing, as a proportion of time spent racing and training, has much the same effect. As the contour of the road rises the cyclist may adapt by changing to a lower gear and increasing pedal rate, but as we all know, as the road rises you inevitably must stand on the pedals and grind. Climbing by its nature means higher power output with lower cadence.

Muscle balance

We have examined the position on the bike and discussed how the type of pedals may affect the alignment of the kneecap, but the muscles acting on the kneecap clearly have a profound effect on the patella alignment. Any imbalance in the forces acting on the kneecap may tend to draw the patella out of its natural groove. Any imbalance in the strength of the muscle groups on the front of the thigh may have a profound affect. The quadriceps muscle group on the thigh is composed of four muscles. Perhaps the most important of these is the muscle group on the inside or medial side known as vastus medialis and in particular the component known as vastus medialis obliquus. The lower fibres of this muscle, vastus medialis obliquus, join the kneecap just at the top of the kneecap on the inside, and can be demonstrated by tensing the thigh muscle. As you can see this is the only muscle on the inside acting against the other three components which make up the remainder of the muscle. If this muscle is weakened in any way it is easy to see how the kneecap could be drawn out of its natural groove.

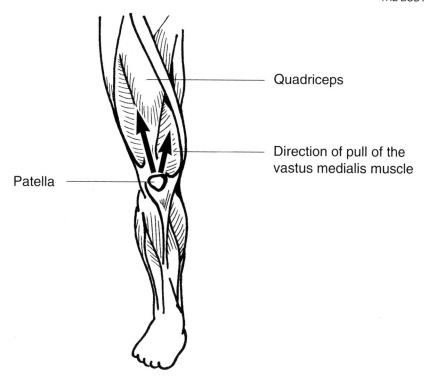

Quadriceps

Direction of pull of the
vastus medialis muscle

Patella

Unfortunately this particular muscle is very prone to weakening or atrophy. The medical term for this weakening is 'wasting' and wasting of the vastus medialis occurs very early in any knee injury. Thus any minor knee injury may cause some wasting. It is of great importance when recommencing training after a knee injury that you should try to ensure adequate retraining of the quadriceps. Returning to training without sufficient rehabilitation may provoke further long term knee pain. Rehabilitation must emphasise retraining of vastus medialis obliquus.

Quadriceps muscle training
It is clearly of fundamental importance to maintain the strength of this muscle group. The traditional weight training exercises used to strengthen the quadriceps such as squats and leg extension exercises may be of minimal benefit. The muscle fibres of vastus medialis obliquus are used mostly in the last 15 degrees of extension or the last part of the leg straightening. This movement is not trained well in the traditional lower limb weight training exercises.

Appropriate exercises may be static or dynamic. The appropriate static exercises are known as 'quads drill'. With the leg straight, tighten the muscles to pull on the kneecap. Try to pull on the kneecap as hard as possible using the muscles on the front of the thigh. Follow the rule of tens: hold the contraction for ten seconds, relax for ten seconds and do this ten times. Quads drill is the exercise most likely to be taught to a patient in hospital after knee surgery.

Dynamic exercises are those which involve movement, for example lifting weights. It is important to remember that even in dynamic exercise the muscle contraction should be with the leg in no greater than 15 degrees of bend in order to train the most important part of the muscle.

Hold the leg over the end of a weight bench in 15 degrees of flexion and extend the leg, using light weights of no more than two pounds initially. This exercise may be easily done at home by training the leg over the end of the bed with a carrier bag with some weights such as books etc.

A combination of these is the 'squeeze pillow' exercise. Sit in bed with a pillow under the slightly bent leg. Try to squeeze the pillow as hard as possible with the back of the leg.

Coping with knee pain

With minor degrees of knee pain the cyclist may continue to train on the bike but there are some important modifications to the training. Lower your saddle. Cycle only on the level and at high cadence with no excess stress. No climbing. Climbing inevitably means a lower cadence with greatly increased forces on the kneecap. If you have introduced extra long cranks then go back to your old ones. If you ride cleats then you are best advised to go back to the traditional clips and straps, perhaps even without shoe plates at least in the beginning, so that your foot may adjust itself freely to its natural position. Stay off your knees as much as possible. If you are a plumber or electrician (or clergyman!) this may be difficult, otherwise leave the gardening or carpet laying to someone else.

Do not race or time trial. We are all competitive, that's why we are racing cyclists, but it is impossible to race and protect your knee. Only race when the knee is able to cope with a full training load.

Sometimes the doctor will prescribe anti-inflammatory medication. While these may reduce the inflammation at the back of the kneecap they cure only the symptoms and not the cause of the problem.

Think therefore of the cause of the problem and do not use these tablets simply as a means of reducing the pain so you can continue training and racing as before, without making the necessary adjustments to your bike or training programme. Anti-inflammatory medication is now available in the form of a gel or foam which may avoid some of the side effects of the tablets.

Injections

Injection of steroids (corticosteroids, not anabolic steroids!). These injections may reduce inflammation in the joint but they always cause some breakdown of tissue within the joint. Treat the cause. Injection into the joint may be a very short term answer but only stores up greater problems for the future. Injections into the actual knee joint are not recommended.

Surgery

There are many operations described in the treatment of anterior knee pain. Remember that in medicine if there are many different treatments then you can be sure that there is no one treatment that really works well! The message is to avoid surgery. The time spent in surgery, recovery, and rehabilitation may be longer than you would spend if you simply let the inflammation reduce by rest alone then build up training.

The various operations include:

- shaving the posterior surface off the kneecap
- moving the point of insertion of the tendon so that the draw of the muscle is more direct to the top of the leg
- drilling holes in the kneecap, or a combination of these.

If you are a serious cyclist who is absolutely committed to the bike and have had great problems with your knee for a long time then surgery may be the last resort. However there are no guarantees in medicine and you may end back where you started only poorer.

Knee pain is the curse of the cyclist and must be treated seriously. Part of the macho image of cycling is the ability to suffer! Knee pain is not a pain to be suffered, it will only get worse. Treat it seriously and with respect. Look after your body as well as you look after your bike!

Osgood Schlatters

In adolescents pain can occur at the upper part of the tibia bone of the lower leg, just where the tendon of quadriceps is attached to the bone. This is felt as a chronic ache, made worse by cycling and associated with a painful tender swelling just below the knee. This is known as Osgood Schlatter's disease after the doctors who first described it.

Osgood Schlatters is an apophysitis. This means an inflammation of the point where the tendon attaches itself to the bone. In the younger age group the tendon is often stronger than the bone, so with frequent and sustained contraction of the muscle, the tendon can pull on the bony attachment causing inflammation and even occasionally pull the attachment off the bone. It is a very common injury in young cyclists and often occurs at a time when they are most keen and enthusiastic. It is also common in runners and footballers. The treatment is to reduce the stress on the tendon attachment. In effect this means avoiding cycling for a period of time. It is frustrating for the young cyclist who probably sustained the injury because they were so keen and enthusiastic in the first place. However there is no substitute for rest. This means rest only from the types of sport that cause it. In order to maintain cardiovascular fitness the cyclist should really attempt to maintain an aerobic sport and the most appropriate sport in these circumstances is swimming.

Hamstring tendinitis

The hamstring muscles are the group of muscles at the back of the leg extending from the buttock to the knee. If you feel behind your knee you will find two firm bands of tissue from the muscle extending across the back of the knee. These form a cup at the back of your knee, and are the tendons of the hamstring. They are attached to the bones of the lower leg thus when they tighten they bend your knee. Tendinitis is felt as a chronic irritating pain in these tendons. They are tender to squeeze and rub. Tendinitis occurs as an overuse injury and may be associated with an increase in training, racing or during a stage race. The treatment is ice and massage. Topical anti-inflammatory creams are of some benefit and oral anti-inflammatory tablets can also be of benefit. The onset of this pain may be associated with a change in bike position but is usually mainly due to an increase in intensity of exercise.

This type of injury is most common when you rotate your leg during the pedal stroke. It is thus more common where there is a biomechanical abnormality of the leg, such as leg length difference or flat feet. In the presence of these minor anomalies we make subconscious adjustments to our pedalling technique. With increases in mileage or intensity of exercise, the excess stress on local structures due to these minor abnormalities can become a source of weakness. The excess stress may be manifest in tendinitis. If in addition you use clipless pedals, where the mobility of the foot is very restricted then your body's capacity to cope with minor adjustments of posture is reduced, and stress overuse reactions are more common.

Hamstring tendinitis is felt as an aching pain along the tendon. There may be some swelling and tenderness of the body of the tendon. The condition should be treated as with any anti-inflammatory reaction, ie with rest, ice, anti-inflammatory tabs or gel. There should be the appropriate adjustment of technique and pedals if necessary and a gradual period of rehabilitation.

If the condition is allowed to progress to a chronic condition, tender local nodules may form in the tendon itself or at the insertion of the tendon. Occasionally this may be treated by an injection of a small quantity of corticosteroid.

With hamstring tendinitis it is common to develop a relative weakness of the hamstring muscle group. Training for the recovery of strength of this muscle group should be an integral part of rehabilitation, as any strength imbalance may contribute to the return of symptoms when serious training is recommenced.

The feet

The main pressure point on the feet is at the ball of the foot on the pedal spindle on the down stroke. Pressure is transmitted directly to the feet through the very rigid soles of the cycling shoes. This rigidity enables direct transmission of power to the pedal with least loss of kinetic energy in compression of a shoe. If the shoe sole were soft, as in a running shoe, some energy would be lost in compressing the sole of the shoe rather than turning the pedals. In addition, the foot is held tightly to the pedal by a strap across the dorsum of the foot to maintain position on the upstroke. To be effective this strap must be quite tight but may cause compression with resulting numbness and pain in the foot.

Overuse injuries at the foot and ankle are uncommon in cycling. Achilles tendinitis is rare in cyclists compared to runners but does occur.

Achilles tendinitis

Achilles tendinitis or inflammation of the Achilles tendon, affects many athletes, especially those who take part in endurance sports where constant repetitive use of the muscles for long periods may cause pain and inflammation in the tendon. The Achilles tendon is at the lower calf where the muscles, the gastrocnemius and soleus, are attached to the heel bone, the calcaneus, found at the back of the foot.

The early symptom of Achilles tendinitis is a slight stiffness in the early morning which eases during the day. As the condition worsens, there may be pain associated with the stiffness which also eases as the day wears on. This pain may also come on during exercise. In these early stages the pain may only be present at the start of exercise, and ease as the exercise progresses.

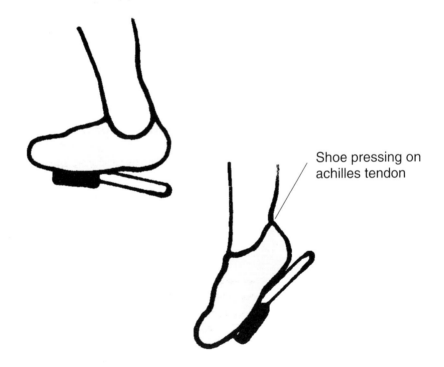

Shoe pressing on achilles tendon

With severe tendinitis, there may be swelling of the Achilles tendon which is most painful during exercise. The tendon will also be swollen and tender to touch.

Footwear is one of the most common factors in bringing on Achilles tendinitis. The Achilles heel tab, found on many cycling and running shoes, is a typical example. Introduced by shoe manufacturers, mainly to make the shoe look good, heel tabs provide a snug fit to the heel when standing, but they may dig into the back of the heel during the pedal revolution. This is more pronounced in cyclists who pedal with their toes pointing down. If you 'toe down' at the lowest part of the pedal revolution, the heel tab will impinge even more on the Achilles tendon.

The treatment in this case is surgery – to the shoe. Cut a semi circle to the back of the shoe, removing the entire heel tab, or cut two slits on either side of the heel tab so that it flops loosely at the back of the shoe. This should ensure that no part of the shoe impinges on your Achilles tendon. Lower the saddle which means you will not toe-down so much at the bottom of the down stroke.

If running is part of the training programme, be sure to wear shoes which are appropriate for the sport. Running shoes should offer adequate cushioning and support, but the so-called Achilles protector at the back of the shoe may cause problems. The remedy, once again, is to cut away the heel tab.

Remember also to look at everyday shoes which may also contribute to Achilles tendinitis. Special attention should be paid to training shoes worn casually. Heel tabs on everyday shoes should also be surgically removed.

Wearing a heel raise in sports and daily-wear shoes may help to relieve tension and take some of the stretch off the tendon. The raise be may one half to one centimetre high inserted into the shoe. Heel raises can be purchased in most sports shops.

Physiotherapy may also be of benefit. The treatment is usually a combination of ultra sound, laser treatment and friction massage and stretching exercises.

Nonsteroidal anti-inflammatory drugs (NSAIDs) may help reduce the pain and swelling in the soft tissue. These should be taken with food, as they may cause some stomach upset. NSAIDs should be discontinued if symptoms of intolerance begin.

Some examples of NSAIDs include Brufen, Naprosyn, Lederfen, Feldene and Oruvail. These are usually prescribed by a doctor, although Brufen may be purchased without a prescription under the brand name Nurofen. Don't take Brufen and Nurofen at the same time.

The last resort, before surgery is steroid injection. While these may reduce inflammation, they also cause some weakening of the tissue. Steroid injections are used to treat many soft tissue conditions, but in cases of Achilles tendinitis, special attention is needed. The Achilles tendon carries great loads, especially during sport. Steroid injections give short term relief at a price. They may cause significant weakening of the tendon with possible tendon rupture. Rupture of the Achilles tendon will mean a minimum of eight weeks in plaster, with or without surgery. That's an entire season.

Tibialis anterior tendinitis

Tendinitis may also occur to the tendons at the front of the foot. The muscles at the front of the foot, in particular a muscle named tibialis anterior are used to draw the foot upwards during the pedal revolution. The tendon may become inflamed, especially if the saddle is too high, where the foot must be drawn up more during the upstroke. Tibialis anterior tendinitis is treated, as with any inflammatory tendinitis, by ice and anti-inflammatory medication.

Cramp

Muscle cramp is a sudden involuntary muscle spasm that usually occurs in the calf. It may be acutely painful and the muscle may be seen and felt to stand out. It may occur spontaneously, often at night, for no apparent reason. Muscle spasms may occur occasionally after a long hard race where they are associated with muscle exhaustion and related to dehydration and glycogen depletion. However more often cramps occur for no apparent reason and some individuals appear to be more prone.

Flat feet (Pes Planus)

Flat feet do not harm the efficiency of the pedal stroke. Indeed, compared to runners, cyclists are at considerable advantage in that they may participate and compete without ill effect in spite of marked foot posture problems. Occasionally biomechanical abnormalities may give rise to compensatory rotatory movements at the ankle and knee which can cause pain and discomfort. This is more likely to occur where the feet are held so rigidly that there is no foot mobility. In clipless pedals there is very little movement. Recently manufacturers have developed some rotatory movements in their pedals, at times up to ten degrees. However this movement is in one plane only and although an advance in design, foot movement normally occurs in three dimension. In traditional pedals and straps there is usually sufficient flexibility to allow the foot enough compensatory movement.

Orthotics

Orthotics are shoe inserts which may alter the biomechanics of foot posture and thus alter the transmission of forces generated on the footplate. In some cases of biomechanical abnormality this may ensure the correct transmission of forces to the legs which would otherwise cause injury. Occasionally in anterior knee pain, hamstring tendinitis and Achilles tendinitis, unresponsive to simple medical management, orthotics can offer benefit. Orthotics are usually moulded and fitted by a podiatrist or physiotherapist with special expertise.

Cold feet

Cold and numb toes may be related to foot straps which are too tight across the top of the foot. Although more common in cold weather, excessively tight toestraps can cause the problem in all conditions. If the toestrap is too tight it can restrict blood flow to the forefoot. Lack of blood supply renders the foot cold and numb. It may be eased by relaxing the foot straps or change of type of pedal from the clip and toestrap to the clip-on type.

INJURIES TO THE TRUNK

Back pain

Backache is a feature of cycling from the top professional to the modest veteran. It may threaten the career of the elite or simply spoil the pleasure of the club run. Cyclists often suffer from low back pain and we all recognise that familiar low backache after a long hard ride in a race or training. It is partly due to our position on the bike: the cycling position is ergonomically unsound which means quite simply that we were not meant to fold up in the way we ride our bikes!

Back pain

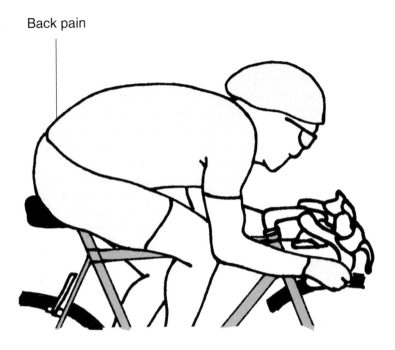

Most low back pain in cyclists is mechanical and ligamentous and is directly related to our position. The cycling position combined with long periods spent racing and training may stress the ligaments of the lower spine especially when our muscles are tired after a long hard ride. It is more likely to recur when riding hard, grinding out the high gears without a break, often into a headwind. With most racing there are periods of relative calm which allow the cyclist to adjust his or her posture, sections of climbing, which allow the cyclist to stand on the pedals or corners where the cyclist must stand up and sprint. These changes of terrain and tempo allow the cyclist to alter posture. However with long races of attrition the back is under constant and unrelenting pressure. It is also important that the cyclist should not be crouched over the top tube but should be able to lengthen out and uncoil. You will note that the top professionals always appear relaxed on their bikes with the pelvis rotated and backs extended, their arms slightly bent to take vibration from the bars and act as shock absorbers.

When we pedal we generate pressure on the pedals by extending the legs using the back as a fixed point. The lower back must cope with this pressure for hours on end, aided only by the back muscles and ligaments so that when the muscles tire the ligaments are relatively unprotected. In most cyclists the back muscles are not well developed. This means that most of the pressure is taken by the ligaments so chronic ligament strain is common. The cyclist may help relieve the pressure from time to time by standing on the pedals, stretching and arching backwards, allowing the muscles to relax for a moment. Remember that during a race you may not be as stable when standing and so lose your line in the bunch, lose the wheel in the line out, or fall and bring others down.

It helps also to improve the flexibility of the lower back. With an inflexible lower spine (ie the lower five vertebrae) you may be unable to lengthen out so instead of conducting pressure through the pelvis to the vertebral bones the ligaments between these bones may be stretched excessively. Hence flexibility is important. Again, cyclists tend to have poor natural flexibility so it is essential that the cyclist work on flexibility not only during training but also throughout the racing season.

The tendency to back pain may also be eased by developing the abdominal muscles. This may seem a little unexpected but remember that when you lift or take pressure on your back it is not simply the back muscles that take the strain but the abdominal muscles also contract which gives the back muscles something to work against for stability.

Cyclists have notoriously bad abdominal muscles. Even cyclists at the top level, who are superbly conditioned endurance athletes, may appear to have 'pot bellies' simply due to poor abdominal muscle tone. Abdominal muscles may be strengthened by performing sit ups. These sit ups should be done with the knees bent. Not only will this improve appearance, but it will also aid muscle balance and posture.

Slipped disc

Occasionally low back pain may be associated with pain down the leg known as Sciatica. This pain may be felt as a shooting or nagging pain along the back of the leg. It may sometimes be associated with weakness of the leg muscles and absence of some of the leg reflexes. These symptoms may be due to what we in layman's terms call a 'slipped disc'. The pain is not actually from the leg but comes from the sciatic nerve which tracks down the leg. The pain is felt along the path of the nerve. Occasionally the nerve affected is the femoral nerve which is the nerve to the front of the thigh. The large bones of the back known as vertebrae each have a piece of gristle or cartilage between them to act as shock absorbers. This is what is commonly known as a disc. The nerves acting on the muscles and providing sensation to the leg come from the spinal cord close to this gristle. Sometimes the gristle may be displaced in such a way that it presses on the nerve. Hence the term slipped disc. Instead of feeling the pain at the point of impingement in the back the body feels this pain as if it came from the leg further down. With a severe problem the treatment is bed rest, to allow the muscle spasm to ease and the pain to subside. This is another occasion where you should certainly not 'ride the pain out' but should be guided by your doctor. Disc problems are very slow to clear and often recurrent. Sometimes bed rest alone is insufficient to ease a disc problem and surgery may be required. The operation aims to relieve the pressure on the nerve by removing part of the disc and thus ease the leg pain. However it does not treat any underlying back weakness so physiotherapy and exercise post operatively are a fundamental part of the recovery.

When you get the go-ahead to return to training, approach your training with care. Cycle first on flat roads, take it easy and look closely at your flexibility. Increase the mileage and intensity very gradually and stop whenever any pain or discomfort returns. Rushing the return to a previous level of fitness is only likely to cause long term problems.

Stress fractures

Stress fractures of the back, while being a common sports injury in general are relatively rare in cycling. Stress fractures occur where the back is used in weight bearing, usually in sports where the back is hyperextended such as gymnastics and butterfly swimming. This type of injury is most unlikely to occur under the normal course of cycle racing and training!

However, stress fractures may occur with weight training. Some weight training programmes include heavy weights in the squats and powerclean exercises. It is vitally important to develop good weight lifting technique, use the most suitable equipment and partake only in supervised training when using heavy weights. Backache while weight training is an important symptom. Do not persist with weight training if suffering from back problems.

The older cyclist

Low back pain is more likely to occur in the older cyclist. The older cyclist is often not as well able to 'spin' and may rely greatly on high gears. Combined with less flexibility and perhaps a degree of the normal wear and tear of the passing years, the older cyclist may find chronic ligament pain a particular problem. The mature cyclist with backache should look very closely at other aspects of lifestyle including the normal technique of lifting, spending long periods in the car, and the various postures adopted in every day work and at home. It often helps to raise the handlebars some centimetres to avoid the need for great flexibility. What is lost in aerodynamics may be gained in comfort!

GROIN INJURIES

Certain conditions may cause problems in the groin area, especially in male cyclists. With apologies to female readers this section deals more closely with problems that affect males!

There are a number of groin problems that occur simply due to the nature of the sport, through spending long periods sitting in the saddle. You sit astride the saddle with the body weight on two bony points known as the ischial tuberosities, covered by muscle and fat. Because cyclists train and race for long periods, these pressure points may become inflamed causing pain due to compression and friction. Saddle soreness, which we have almost all experienced, is an inflammation of the subcutaneous tissues. It has a medical name acute panniculitis. With continued friction and weight bearing, the condition may worsen causing more serious damage to the fat pad, and a condition known as fat necrosis. Friction is reduced by wearing seamless shorts with elastic leg openings. The crotch of the shorts should be of chamois or a synthetic reproduction which cyclists often lubricate with Vaseline or lanolin. With cycle races lasting three or four hours, the crotch becomes hot and sticky, so groin hygiene is especially important to avoid infection. Infection may produce folliculitis with boils or abscesses and these require medical treatment.

Haemorrhoids, commonly called piles, are unpleasant and uncomfortable. Thrombosed external haemorrhoids are an especially nasty variant. These occur as a sudden painful swelling at the anus with a lump that looks like a black grape. If you have a thrombosed external haemorrhoid you will be unable to sit down and, needless to say, this condition requires medical attention.

Torsion of the testis.

Cyclists rarely wear undergarments as it is more comfortable to wear only cycling shorts. The scrotum, containing the testicles, hangs loose in the groin. The testicle, which is hanging loose in the scrotum only supported by the blood vessels and spermatic cord, may occasionally twist on itself. If this happens, then the blood supply may be cut off and without blood supply for any significant length of time the testicle may be damaged and this may harm fertility. Torsion of the testis is painful and this pain may be felt in the scrotum, but may also be felt in the loin or side and make you nauseous. If an athlete, in any sport, or indeed any male, complains of persistent pain in the testicle it is important to seek help immediately because it may require urgent surgery to save the testicle. Thankfully this is a relatively rare condition.

Numbness in the groin.

The pressure from sitting on the saddle for long period of time may bruise or damage the structures of the perineum between the scrotum and the anus. This pressure may bruise a nerve called the ilioinguinal nerve, which is the sensory nerve supply to the scrotum and penis. This neuropraxia or nerve bruising will cause numbness. To avoid this nerve bruising you should stand up or at least shift your position in the saddle from time to time to prevent nerve bruising.

Priapism

Priapism is a most alarming phenomenon which has been noted to occur in cyclists. Priapism is a painful persistent erection but it is very rare. It is a condition that would certainly gain attention and is easily remembered! In theory it may occur through a badly fitting saddle putting pressure on the pudendal nerve. Medical help should be sought.

Hernias

A hernia is commonly known as a rupture. It occurs where part of the abdominal wall is weakened and allows some of the abdominal contents to swell out like a balloon under the skin. A hernia can occur in anyone but is more likely in those who lift heavy loads at work or who do weight training. While it may cause discomfort and occasionally pain, the main worry is that the contents of this hernia sac become trapped and/or their blood supply is impaired. When this occurs we call it strangulation of the hernia and it may cause severe pain and permanent damage. It is advised that most hernias should be repaired by surgery. Most hernia operations are done in a one-day procedure so that you are back home very quickly, but you would be well advised to rest afterwards for up to six weeks. Any increase abdominal pressure by weight training, intensive exercise while racing or even with a severe cough may weaken the repair.

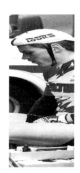

CHAPTER 4

THE MUSCLES

The main muscle activity of cycling occurs through movement at the ankle, knee, and hip and in the sustained use of muscles across these joints. Each pedal revolution requires sequential and co-ordinated dynamic activity of these main muscle groups. Other muscle groups are used, but mostly to stabilise the body to ensure efficient use of the dynamic muscles. Posture is maintained by the fixed contraction of other major muscle groups and this type of muscle contraction is known as an isometric contraction.

The pedalling movement commences with the downstroke through leg extension. The knee is straightened through the activity of those muscles on the front of the thigh, the quadriceps group combined with hip extension through the action of the gluteals, the muscles of the buttocks. Straightening the upper leg at the hip joint, known as hip extension, occurs by contraction of gluteus maximus, the main muscle of the buttock, with some contribution from the hamstrings, the muscles at the back of the leg. Gluteus maximus is active mostly in the first 45 degrees of extension. The hamstrings are active in the last 45 degrees and continue to draw through 180 degrees and the initial upstroke.

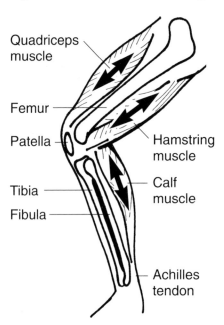

Quadriceps muscle

Femur

Patella

Tibia

Fibula

Hamstring muscle

Calf muscle

Achilles tendon

Straightening the leg at the knee, known as knee extension, occurs by the action of the quadriceps group through a 70-degree revolution. The quadriceps is made up of four main muscles, the three muscles of the vasti group and rectus femoris. These are active to 15 degrees through the horizontal. This extensor movement continues at the ankle by pushing the front part of the foot downwards, known as plantar flexion, through the action of the gastrocnemius and soleus, the calf muscles, on the down stroke. On the upstroke the muscle used to pull the front of the foot upwards is known as tibialis anterior. There should not be any rocking or sideways movement at the ankle joint, inversion or eversion.

One of the two calf muscles crosses the back of the knee, the gastrocnemius. It helps to bend the knee assisted by the hamstrings. Flexion, the medical term for bending, of the hips occurs using muscles at the front of the hip joint called psoas and iliacus.

During this time the trunk is held firm by the large muscle groups of the back and the abdominal muscles. The activity of muscles and the order in which they contract has been studied in great detail using electrical sensors known as electromyography or EMG. The activity of each muscle during the pedal revolution has been analysed to demonstrate how the activities of all the muscle groups dovetail to allow the smooth activity of each pedal revolution.

It is interesting to note the effect of alterations in saddle height on electrical or EMG activity; it shows that changes in saddle height can alter the balance of the muscle activity. Rectus femoris was found to be more active at a lower saddle height of 95% leg length, while raising the saddle height to 105% leg length increased the activity of another muscle known as sartorius. At lower saddle height greater activity was noted in quadriceps femoris. Saddle height may also be a factor in knee injury and cyclists tend to suffer anterior knee pain if the saddle is too high. Variation in saddle height alters muscle balance and this may be a possible causative factor.

Many studies have tried to determine the most efficient cycling posture. One study found that cycling on the drops resulted in much more effective oxygen use, easier breathing and more work output. They were not concerned with aerodynamics, but simply power and work output and they emphasised that posture was crucial for optimal performance. Other work has also shown that improvements in riding style may improve efficiency. Posture is important also in eliminating drag. Wind resistance or aerodynamic drag increases greatly as speed increases; and in mathematical terms it has been shown that aerodynamic drag increases as the square on the velocity increases.

Cycling position and posture attract great attention in cycling coaching theory. Scientific investigation confirms the coaching principles that position and posture may greatly influence your ability to achieve your physiological potential.

PHYSIOLOGY

Cycling is represented across the spectrum of physiological performance. Within cycling we have two extremes of performance from short track sprints lasting just over ten seconds to the multi stage tours such as the Tours of France, Italy, and Spain, each lasting several weeks with stages well over 100 miles, and climbing some of Europe's highest mountain passes. Different types of performance are required in various stages or even within each stage, from the mass sprint in a flat stage, to the sustained climbing in the mountains.

Most leisure cycling and cycle touring is of a sustained nature and fits the classic definition of aerobic or endurance sport. Cycle sprinting is quite specialised and has very different physiological requirements, but we shall concentrate on the endurance aspects of the sport.

Through scientific study of elite cyclists we have developed a good understanding of the physiological qualities necessary to be a top class performer. There are two main ways in which muscles can work known as aerobic and anaerobic. Cycling demands high aerobic capacity to cope with the sustained, relatively high intensity workload. Aerobic capacity is the ability to breathe and use oxygen efficiently and is the essential quality in all endurance sport. Exceptional anaerobic tolerance is necessary to cope with the surges required to escape from the peloton or to chase a breakaway. Anaerobic capacity is the ability to sprint hard without matching the effort in breathing. Anaerobic effort produces lactic acid and anaerobic tolerance is the ability to cope with increased lactic acid levels. An elite cyclist therefore has relatively high aerobic capacity, as represented by VO_2 max, but also has high lactate tolerance and ability to perform while coping with lactate load.

An elite cyclist also has little excess weight and so has a low body fat percentage (male 6–9% and female 12–15%). Elite cyclists will also have good quadriceps muscle strength and local muscle endurance.

Cycling is an endurance sport with the body weight supported in contrast to running where body weight is carried. Body weight may be seen as unimportant but in most cycling events there is an uphill component, during which time gravity draws against the forward motion of the body. Going uphill it would be best to be as small and light as possible. On the other hand, the smaller the cyclist the smaller the engine! Climbing is thus very specialised and to be an efficient climber you must be as fit as possible but also as light as possible. In scientific terms we can appreciate that it is not enough to have a large engine, expressed in terms of VO_2 max, but aerobic capacity related to body weight is the critical guide to performance potential. This is known as the power to weight ratio and is well illustrated in the body configuration, known as somatotype, of elite cyclists. Climbers tend to have low body weight while true time trialists and pursuiters have greater muscle bulk. True sprinters tend to be of similar size and shape to power athletes and athletic sprinters, but tend to be poor climbers and moderate pursuiters. The exaggerated body shape of the various team specialists in an event such as the Tour of France is reflected in their performance: sprinters tend to have difficulty in the mountains, and the climbers are seldom seen contesting the sprints. All rounders fit roughly in between! The winner in an event such as the Tour of France will have the ideal talent mix in all areas – Miguel Indurain is a classic example.

In many sports your ability to perform is inherited from your parents. This is especially true in endurance sports. There are interesting parallels in animal sports, where horses, dogs and even pigeon breeds are considered so important that vast sums are invested in buying animals with the correct pedigree without any indication of ability or performance.

An endurance athlete requires a high oxygen uptake capacity (VO_2 max) coupled with the appropriate muscle fibre type distribution. Various studies on training and performance of athletes in many sports have shown that the potential for improvement in VO_2 max is limited. Maximum improvements are unlikely to be greater than 10% to 15%. In order to be an elite performer the more successful cyclist must have inherited aerobic capacity which is considerably above average values. The oxygen uptake profile for top performance has been estimated from the examination of many of elite cyclists. The average values needed to excel range from 67 ml/kg/min to 74 ml/kg/min and these values compare very favourably with established values for elite athletes in other endurance sports.

Although investigation of elite cyclists demonstrates consistently high values for VO_2 max, which seem essential for elite performance, it is interesting to note one study where there was an attempt to predict 25-mile time trial results based on parameters of physiological assessment. The best indicator of cycling performance was found, not to be VO_2 max or aerobic capacity, but to be cycling experience. There is clearly more to performance than VO_2 max!

So what does determine the difference in performance amongst the good and the top performers while values for aerobic capacity are broadly similar? As with other endurance sports it is often not so much the ability to produce a maximal performance which may be reflected in VO_2 max, but efficiency of performance at various submaximal levels of exertion. It is the relationship between the intensity of exercise and the production of lactic acid, measured as onset of blood lactate, or anaerobic threshold that is important together with efficiency on the bike.

Women's cycling has also reached new heights in popularity. VO_2 max values for female cyclists compare favourably with those for other endurance athletes. The comparable figures for aerobic capacity of female cyclists are 55–65 mls/kg/min.

Scientific testing

Scientific testing may give some guidance to individual physiological capacity which may then be compared to the top performers. More importantly, it allows an athlete and their coach to compare performance and training over a period of time and adjust training as appropriate. It is essential when measuring physiological parameters of elite cyclists that the type of test protocol and the testing equipment mimic the type of performance and the cycle used in racing. Ideally the actual racing cycle normally ridden should be used on a weighted roller or on a treadmill. The most common testing rig, is a weighted roller gaining resistance from a wind fan. Such a test rig, constructed to simulate the sport, is called an ergometer.

Do not be convinced by VO_2 max studies that do not use a bicycle. Values measured using a running treadmill or an exercise bicycle, not identical to the racing bike, do not give comparable results. Various studies have examined performance on cycle ergometers and treadmill running, and found VO_2 max determined on a cycling ergometer to be as much as 10% less than when running. These studies did not use specialised cyclists. Endurance trained cyclists were found to have VO_2 max and anaerobic threshold values greater than on treadmill running. The important message is that testing should be done to simulate the sport.

Heart rate monitors are increasingly used by cyclists in training but to get the best use from the monitors, heart rates equivalent to VO_2 max and anaerobic threshold should be determined experimentally. These should then be used to set target heart rates. By using training heart rate targets cyclists can focus training to improve particular aspects of performance. Heart rates can be used to establish target bands for oxidative metabolic training and to establish adequate recovery in interval training. Anaerobic threshold usually occurs at 70–85% of VO_2 max, depending on the athletes state of physiological training and this heart rate is used in sustained interval training. Target rates of 60–70% maximum are used as target bands for long distance oxidative training.

Cadence

Cycling cadence describes the rate of pedal revolution. Cycling lore, and the various coaching manuals, emphasise high pedalling cadence. Indeed, the accepted mark of the elite cyclist is the ability to 'spin'. This phenomenon interested scientists who were initially unable to demonstrate improved efficiency at these higher cadences and indeed earlier studies suggested that the optimal cycling cadence should be much lower than that normally utilised by elite cyclists. Looking at other sports we find that rowers use an optimal stroke rate of approximately 34 strokes per minute and cross country skiers likewise a low slide rate.

These early studies were however performed on non specialist cyclists, however, unskilled cyclists use different muscles than experienced cyclists when cycling at high rates. The better studies which used experienced cyclists found that faster cycling rate has a smaller oxygen cost to the elite cyclist, so there does appear to be a significant advantage in maintaining a higher cadence. Cycling efficiency is so specific that variations in aerobic and anaerobic threshold parameters have even been demonstrated on cyclists wearing toeclips or cleated shoes.

MUSCLE FIBRE TYPE

Muscle fibre type has a large part to play in determining natural ability in cycling. Some of us are born endurance athletes and some of us are born with a natural talent in sprinting. Muscle fibre type determines this natural ability. Of course, we may train to optimise an inherent ability or to compensate for any lack of natural ability but genetic potential has a very important role.

You may have been born to thunder up the Champs Elysee, drive past the lead-out wheel and take the chequered flag arms aloft. On the other hand, you may be destined for the lone break of 100k, working long and hard to finish alone, celebrating along the finishing straight minutes ahead of the peloton. Perhaps, you are a born track sprinter or your speed endurance makes you better suited for the team time trial. Unfortunately, though many of us may dream of accepting the bouquet on the podium, many of us are simply not made for this stardom. Renowned sprinters were born with this natural ability that others do not possess. Being a top sprinter isn't easy because that talent must be nurtured, trained, and honed to perfection. While born with the raw material, only hours of training and preparation can develop and refine that talent.

What is a sprinter? A sprinter has the ability to accelerate and maintain great speed for a short burst. This may be the final sprint in a stage race or the short burst of the track sprint. It is sheer speed and the sprint is anaerobic. This means that the sprinter races flat out, and afterwards gasps for breath. The body has not been able to supply enough oxygen for muscle activity, the muscle burns energy without oxygen and must pay it back later. This is known as oxygen debt.

The endurance cyclist, on the other hand, has the ability to maintain high speed for a sustained period of time. This type of rider may be particularly suited to a high speed lone break, not at the maximum speed of the sprinter but a sustained high speed for a much longer period of time. At the end of this effort they are not gasping for breath, because they have been able to breathe enough oxygen during the event to feed the muscles.

What is this natural talent that makes a top sprinter and why are there lone break specialists? The answer is in analysis of the muscle. We all recognise natural ability. Behind it is a complex physiological machine that is specially tuned to perform in a particular manner. It is the of the muscle to contract at speed that creates the sprinter and, for an endurance event, performance is limited by the endurance capacity of the muscles involved in those particular movements. Not all muscle is the same and, at the limit, performance is determined by very specialised forms of muscle. Scientists have identified two basic types of muscle fibre known as fast twitch and slow twitch. Fast twitch muscle has a particular ability to contract at high speed and has adapted to provide the energy needed for this very rapid muscle contraction without oxygen. This energy supply although rapid, is not very efficient and only works for a very short period of time. It produces a waste product known as lactic acid.

We all know about lactic acid and we recognise that we cannot sprint indefinitely as muscles become stiff, sore and seize up. It is the increasing acidity due to the lactic acid that slows up the muscles. On the other hand, slow twitch muscle fibres have developed an ability to continue contracting almost indefinitely, not as rapidly as the fast twitch but providing there is enough oxygen and energy available slow twitch muscles can continue to work almost indefinitely. Not unexpectedly these are the muscle fibres most suited to endurance.

When scientists test the muscles of the top sprinters and endurance athletes of all sportsmen and sportswomen, not just cycling, a pattern emerges. Endurance athletes, such as long distance cyclists, runners, rowers and cross-country skiers have a greater proportion of slow twitch fibres. Sprinters, power athletes and jumpers have a greater proportion of fast twitch fibres. Muscle fibre type can be established by biopsy where a small piece is taken from the muscle and examined under a microscope. A small sliver of muscle, approximately the dimensions of a match stick, but only one third the length is removed using a large bore needle under local anaesthetic. Fibre type is determined by staining which colours the fibre types differently. The aerobic, or type one, stain red and the anaerobic, type two, stain white. Hence we hear the terms red and white fibres.

One would assume that a good endurance athlete would have a large proportion of red fibre type, and indeed this is usually the case. The sprinter generally has a large proportion of white fibre type. Could we then predict which athlete would have the potential to be a specialist? In theory this is possible but in practice prediction is not as clear cut. We can tell the slow twitch and fast twitch fibres and know that fast twitch are three times faster than slow twitch but we cannot tell exactly how fast they are, and YOUR slow twitch may be faster than MY fast twitch! There is some predictive value but not enough to be absolutely certain.

It is interesting to note that the fibre types associated with speed and power are similar. This can be seen in practice where power athletes, ie shot putters, discus throwers etc, are often quite good sprinters in spite of their size. This is often demonstrated in club athletic competition where power athletes make up the extra person in the relay event. Muscle fibre type has a great influence on performance in sport but one is born with a certain proportion of muscle fibre type: it is genetic. This cannot be changed, so you are either born with natural ability or without. All is not lost however as you can make the most of your potential and while muscle fibre type cannot be changed from type 1 to type 2, muscles may be trained to improve their efficiency in both aerobic and anaerobic sport. You may not be a born sprinter but you can improve your sprint and develop your speed to a greater extent and even if you may have the muscle fibre type of the sprinter you can improve your endurance. After all, you must improve your endurance ability sufficiently to be able to make it to the finish to use that lethal sprint!

There are three subgroups within the type two fast twitch fibres: 2a, 2b, and 2c. Type 2a fibres can be trained to have some aerobic ability, so endurance training can improve the endurance potential of some fast twitch fibres. With a large proportion of slow twitch fibres you are unlikely ever to be a successful sprinter but you can improve the performance of what you have. Speed of contraction of a muscle is not simply due to the percentage of muscle fibre types but is more closely related to the surface area occupied by these fibre types. Thus through training, although you cannot increase the numbers of each fibre, the fibre enlarges and increases the surface area so you can therefore improve your sprinting ability. You often hear how the stronger endurance riders try to 'ride the sprint out of the sprinters legs' and there is an interesting physiological background to this practical advice.

When you are exercising for a long period such as in a road race, you use slow twitch fibres first. As the speed and intensity of a race increases the body recruits more muscle fibres, and as the intensity continues to increase, you trigger fast twitch fibres to cope with the high load. If a sprinter can ride along in the peloton out of the wind, not taking a turn at the front, he can survive using only slow twitch fibres. If he is in a small breakaway, or forced to the front he must compete at a higher intensity, recruiting fast twitch fibres and producing lactic acid. If he can make it to the finish and tolerate the lactic acid, then when it comes to the sprint these fast twitch fibres are already exhausted and that lethal sprint is neutralised. On the other hand the athlete with the higher proportion of slow twitch fibres can compete at high intensity much longer so these cyclists should try to make it as hard as possible, for as long as possible to eliminate the sprinters. A cycle race thus becomes a game of physiological poker.

What does this mean to you?

The theory is fascinating and scientists continue to unravel the mysteries of human performance. New tests are discovered, new methods of assessment, new measurements of performance but there is only one test of interest to you and me – who crosses the line first? With all the advances in cell chemistry and enzymatic assays there has been little change in the nuts and bolts of training and racing. An athlete may be born with natural ability but that is only part of the jigsaw of successful racing. Even if you are born with natural ability you must train to realise that potential and even if you are not born with a great deal of ability you can still train to make the most of your potential.

You will know yourself, without a biopsy whether you are a sprinter or an endurance athlete and while you must develop your strengths you must try to work on your weaknesses. That is why Greg LeMond is such a good all rounder. Why Sean Kelly, although a renowned sprinter, is a competent time trialist and why Hinault remains a legend.

CHAPTER 5

STRETCHING EXERCISES

Stretching has become an integral part of preparation for racing and training in many sports. It is promoted as a means of preventing injury and as an essential component of rehabilitation after injury. Efforts to highlight the importance of stretching have been so successful that it has achieved importance beyond its true value! Stretching will not make you a faster cyclist by itself and its importance must be kept in perspective. Where it may be of benefit is in helping to prevent injury and by, reducing muscle aches and pains, may enable you to train longer, train harder, and thus improve performance. Stretching therefore should form a regular part of preparation before training and is an essential component of any warm-down routine.

Stretching offers benefits not only when training on the bike but also during winter training, weight training, and after periods of running. Winter weight training uses muscle groups that cyclists neglect for the other nine months of the year; also, training with heavy weights, while increasing strength, increases muscle size and tends to shorten muscles. Increase in muscle bulk known as hypertrophy, may impose inflexibility. Athletes who do regular and frequent heavy weight training tend to become tight and muscle bound unless complementing their training with an adequate stretching programme.

Running is a very different muscle action to cycling with sudden contraction and jarring of the muscle with each stride. It is traumatic, causing muscle soreness and stiffness due to the constant trauma. This muscle soreness, pain and stiffness is partly due to microscopic muscle damage. Unless there is adequate warm down and stretching these aches and pains can remain for some hours or even days after running and prevent further training sessions.

Those who run consistently as part of their training learn to cope with these aches and pains and adapt to the constant trauma. Muscles most likely to become painful are the calf muscles, the soleus and gastrocnemius, and the muscles on the back of the thigh: the hamstring muscles. If running on hills the muscle on the front of the thigh, the quadriceps, may also suffer. Running may shorten muscle, and shortened muscles are more likely to tear when suddenly stretched during sport, for example during the sudden stretching in a sprint. Muscle tears may be prevented by stretching the muscle both before and after each session. After training, it is important to warm down. So, jog for four to five minutes at a much slower pace, breathing easily but maintaining muscle temperature. Muscle recovers from intense activity by removing waste products including lactic acid for redistribution and disposal and this occurs during the warm down. Appropriate stretching exercises in this case are hamstring and calf stretches.

CALF STRETCH

Calf stretching may be performed in a number of different ways: you may stand, leaning against a wall, with your legs outstretched. By relaxing the arms, tension will be felt in the calf. When the muscle is stretched, hold for ten seconds and then relax for ten seconds. A further development of stretching is to make use of the extra

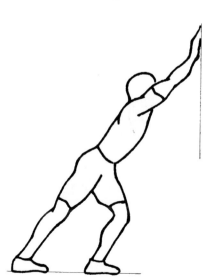

relaxation that occurs in a muscle immediately after contraction. Contract the muscle first relax and then stretch. The extra muscle relaxation after a contraction known as compensatory relaxation. A suitable stretching technique that makes best use of this relaxation would be as follows: tense the muscle for ten seconds, then relax and stretch for ten seconds. It is simply making use of the phase of relaxation immediately after a contraction when relaxation is greatest and the muscle can be stretched more effectively.

HAMSTRINGS

The hamstring muscle is the large muscle group at the back of the thigh which pulls from the bottom to the back of the knee. This muscle is important in cycling, not only because it tends to shorten through the action of pedalling, but because tight hamstrings may be related to low back pain. The hamstring group may be stretched by sitting on the floor and stretching out or by putting the foot of a chair, table or height and stretching.

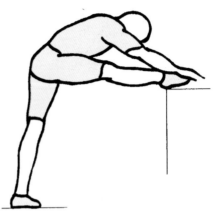

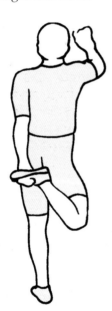

QUADS STRETCH

The quadriceps muscle is the muscle at the front of the thigh. It may be stretched by standing on one leg and pulling the other up behind. Stand, grasping the foot and draw it up behind the bottom. You may feel the tightness as the muscle is drawn taut at the front of the thigh.

ADDUCTORS

The adductors may be stretched by putting the leg up sideways on a chair and gradually stretching out.

BACK

It is very important for cyclists to stretch the lower back especially after a long training spin. Flexibility of the lower back is critical in prevention of low back pain in cyclists. Considerable pressure rises vertically from the pedal spindle and, as the back is stretched across the top tube, these pressures may cause chronic ligamentous low back strain.

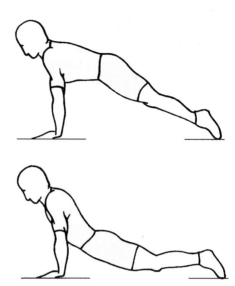

When standing, rotate the trunk. Increase the size of the arc described by the trunk which helps improve all-round mobility. More specific exercises for low back flexion and extension may be performed on the floor. Take a position as if you are about to do a press up. Arch the back forming a large bridge, hold for ten seconds and then return to the normal position. Then reverse the movement by bending back the shoulders, neck and back so the stomach brushes the floor. Hold for ten seconds and repeat.

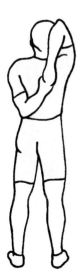

SHOULDERS

There are a number of shoulder mobility and stretching exercises. A typical exercise would be to shrug the shoulders and rotate the shoulder throughout the range of movement by drawing circles with the arms.

A further exercise would be to put one hand behind you back reaching upwards, and the other over the top of the shoulder, and try to join them. Hold and stretch for ten seconds. This exercise is repeated using the arms alternately.

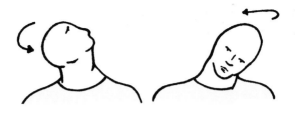

NECK

Neck mobility and flexibility are essential to prevent the aches and pains that occur through wearing hard shell helmets. Chronic neck pain may also occur through the neck extension that is necessary to look forward when you are stretched along the top tube.

Rotate your neck by drawing circles with your head. Increase the arc to increase mobility. Move the neck throughout the range of movement. Bend the neck forward so the chin reaches the chest and then bend the neck backwards. Bend the neck to one side so the ear is close to the shoulder and then to the other side. Rotate the neck as if to look over the shoulder and repeat on the other side.

Care! Older cyclists should be careful when doing these neck mobility exercises as they occasionally cause dizziness or lightheadedness.

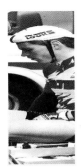

CHAPTER 6

HYGIENE

There are some conditions that can affect the unsuspecting cyclist, which are usually preventable through good hygiene habits. However it has to be recognised that some people are more prone to certain conditions than others. If you are one of these you should be especially particular.

ATHLETES FOOT (TINEA PEDIS)

Athletes foot is a fungal infection of the web space between the toes. The main complaint may be of itchy toes and it occurs particularly between the fourth and fifth toes, though sometimes between the third and fourth. In more severe infections the skin may become soggy, macerated and may split with pain and tenderness. Mild infection may cause irritation and itch, whereas more severe forms may be acutely painful. Mild forms respond to dusting with an antifungal powder, but more severe infection requires treatment with anti fungal creams similar to those used for groin infections. Athletes foot is often spread through communal showers and is made worse by the hot sweaty sticky conditions of a cycling shoe. As part of the treatment of severe infections you should bathe your feet twice daily in a basin of warm water, with just a pinch of salt, dry them thoroughly and apply antifungal cream. Your feet should then be kept clean and dry in clean socks, preferably cotton.

BOILS

An infected boil or abscess may expand causing pain, discomfort and redness in the groin. Your doctor may wish to lance or incise it in his surgery or treatment room. Minor infections may need antibiotic treatment alone and you should avoid the temptation to lance the boil yourself under less than ideal conditions. Large infected abscesses need hospital treatment as these infections may progress to form very nasty infected areas which are very difficult to treat. They may progress to become a chronic infection, forming a pilonidal abscess or sinus. This chronic infection is notoriously difficult to completely cure and may go on to cause problems throughout your cycling career with intermittent swelling, inflammation and discharge. Prevention is the key.

Lancing a boil or abscess should almost always be performed by a doctor in a clinical setting although in exceptional circumstances this may not be possible. If the boil or abscess has burst or has been lanced the pus should be allowed to drain freely. It usually takes four to five days for an abscess to stop draining and the infection to clear. Ideally pressure on the area should be avoided, but most cyclists will be frustrated at not being able to train and wish to return to the bike earlier. If the area remains painful, inflamed and discharging pus it is essential to seek medical assistance. Infections in this area can be persistent and very difficult to treat.

FUNGAL INFECTIONS (TINEA CRURIS)

Many athletes in various sports suffer from fungal groin infections. These infections are so well recognised in the sporting community that they have become known by folk names such as Jock Itch, Crotch Rot etc. They are the groin equivalent of athletes foot! Fungal infection causes a red itchy rash in the groin often spreading to the anal area. It is red, sometimes scaly, and more inflamed at the edges. It forms a continuous red rash which is usually seen at the side of each testicle in men. In women it may sometimes be associated with vaginal thrush infections. The treatment is simple, painless and relatively quick and, although you may be embarrassed and worried that it is something more serious, it is a common infection, and easily treated. The appropriate treatment, an antifungal cream, will be prescribed by your doctor and usually applied twice or three times daily for about one week.

GROIN INFECTION

In our sport we spend considerable time sitting in the saddle, and inevitably the groin becomes hot, sticky and sweaty. Exercising hard, often in warm weather, presents great potential for infection in the groin and perineal area so it is essential to ensure good hygiene by thorough groin washing and meticulous care of shorts and chamois.

Shorts should be kept clean and changed daily. Traditionalists believe that cyclists should use real chamois in their shorts. Real chamois is however very slow to dry when washed and must be dried carefully. Modern imitation chamois shorts are just as comfortable and yet can be washed frequently in a washing machine and dry almost immediately. If shorts are easily washed and dried, they are more likely to be washed frequently!

As the groin is hot and sweaty it is an ideal growing area for infection and bugs find this hot sticky environment ideal. You should shower as soon as is practical after every race and training session, washing thoroughly with soap and water, and drying well. In the absence of proper hygiene, hair follicles can become inflamed, bacteria may thrive and produce a collection of pus, forming boils, carbuncles and abscesses in the groin. In the early stages of infection, while the area is red, inflamed and painful it is best kept clean and dry. If it becomes very inflamed and angry, an antibiotic may be necessary and this can be prescribed by your doctor. If in doubt seek medical advice early.

SWEAT RASH

One often hears the term sweat rash; originally it was used to describe the prickly heat that occurs in hot climates. It is a form of irritation of the sweat glands. There is no specific treatment, but it is more likely to occur when clothing is made of a fabric that does not allow the skin to 'breathe'. Sweat rash is more likely to occur with synthetic clothing, nylon and close fitting lycra garments. There is no treatment other than to keep cool and change to cotton clothing.

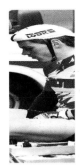

CHAPTER 7

TRAINING

There are many well-recognised essential components of traditional training in cycling. We are all familiar with the terms long slow distance, interval training, sprint training etc. However, the most important principle of training is the specificity of training which means that it must mimic as closely as possible the actual speed and mode of racing. Training must be seen within the context of the sport and aimed towards developing the skills and physiological components of the race itself.

Cycle racing is an endurance sport and as such is built on a broad aerobic base so the greatest part of training must be spent developing this aerobic base. In cycling parlance, we term this 'getting in the miles' and it forms the basis of all training. The traditional weekly club run has grown as a direct result of the need to have at least one long session per week.

There are parallels in other endurance sports such as running, rowing and swimming and one of the greatest ever distance running coaches, Arthur Lydiard, was well known for his maxim that 'mileage makes champions'. Swimmers cover vast mileage throughout their preparation and 'steady state' rowing is the backbone of winter training. Over distance or endurance training is an essential component of all endurance sport and cycling is no different.

HOW DOES TRAINING WORK?

All training is aimed at improving the body's ability to cope with racing. To understand the effects of training we may simplify the effect of training on the body into two components

● The central engine or pump (The heart)

● The transmission (The muscle)

Improvements gained by long distance training occur principally in our muscles, but only in those muscles used during training. Over distance training encourages muscle to adapt to training. Muscle may enlarge a little but most of the changes occur within the muscle itself. Training encourages the development of many microscopic blood vessels within the muscle which are known as capillaries. These small blood vessels feed muscle, so that increasing the network of blood vessels improves supply of oxygen and energy to the muscle.

There are also some improvements within the muscle cell so that better use can be made of the nutrients when they arrive. Special chemicals called enzymes are needed to help use energy in muscle and these are increased by training. The most effective training of muscle occurs at less than maximum training intensity. High intensity exercise generates lactic acid and lactic acid can inhibit the improvements that occur with aerobic training.

It is important to have some guidelines about the frequency and intensity of training: how often to do these long cycles, and how hard. There are many coaching formulae relating exercise intensity to heart rate. All these formulae base the target heart rates on an estimate of maximum heart rate. They make the assumption that maximum heart rate may be calculated by subtracting age in years from 220 (ie 220-age in years, for example a man aged 30 should have a maximum of 190 (220-30=190) These guestimates may be a valid approximation for the average population but for a well trained athlete maximum heart rate may vary greatly. Maximum heart rate may be determined more accurately as follows.

Find a hill that would take between six and 10 minutes to climb at maximum speed. Start off at moderate intensity and gradually increase speed up the hill until going flat out with about two minutes climbing left. Continue at maximum speed and make a special effort about 30 seconds from the top so you have reached absolute maximum. You will probably achieve maximum heart rate on this all-out effort! Use this maximum heart rate to determine the different levels of training. A maximum test should be done when well rested, fresh and enthusiastic. If you are tired and unwilling to give an absolutely maximum effort then your heart rate will not be a true maximum and the entire training programme will be inaccurate.

It is important to emphasise that this maximum all-out effort should only be undertaken by an already very fit young athlete. The older or unfit must not undertake this type of all out effort as its intensity could bring on a myocardial infarction/heart attack in susceptible individuals.

Heart rate is easily measured using a heart rate monitor; they are now relatively inexpensive. If investing in a heart rate monitor, buy a better quality monitor, as an inaccurate monitor is useless for monitoring training intensity precisely. Heart rate may be counted accurately by hand at low rates but is much more difficult as heart rate increases. The pulse at the wrist is found at the fold of the skin, about one or two centimetres from the outside edge with your palm upwards. A stronger pulse and one which is easier to count is felt on the side of the neck. The pulse is usually counted for 15 seconds and multiplied by four.

Scientific protocols are available to determine training intensity to improve performance based on oxygen uptake and lactate level in a laboratory. While laboratory analysis would be ideal, simple heart rate testing can be done by any cyclist and needs no sophisticated equipment. Using heart rate to set training loads gives specific targets for training. The type of training may differ little from usual components of training but using heart rate to regulate training gives a more structured pattern to preparation.

No matter how much we train aerobically this will not prepare us ideally for racing. Although cycling is an endurance sport and a broad aerobic base is essential, when we look at a race pace it is constantly changing. The pace of the bunch varies with surges, bends and rises in the road and for each rider there are constant changes of pace as you maintain your position in the bunch. Cycle racing therefore requires not only an ability to maintain a constant pace, but also the ability to change pace and cope with anaerobic surges. Interval training and sprint training should clearly be an integral part of a planned programme.

Overload and recovery

The basic principle of training is overload and recovery. If we could train consistently above race pace then we could in theory cope better with race pace. Interval training enables us to do this as we train for shorter periods above race pace and recover before starting the next workload. The duration of the training interval is not in itself important and may range from one to ten minutes but the recovery period should be long enough to allow recovery of heart rate to 50% of maximum before beginning the work again. There are many programmes for interval training available from coaching manuals. There is no ideal formula that applies to all cyclists but some examples are shown below. The intervals are periods of high intensity exercise interspersed with periods of rest or low intensity pedalling.

1 One minute on, two minutes off, or two on, one off for 20 minutes,

2 Equal periods of alternating exercise and rest in increments of one, two, three, four, five, four, three, two, one minutes.

3 Three minutes on, one off, two on, one off, three on, one off.

4 Seven minutes on, six off etc.

5 Ten minutes on, five off, ten and five, ten and five etc.

There are many permutations of work periods and rest and no single pattern is best. Unfortunately, interval training may sometimes be difficult to perform on the open road with traffic, changes in terrain, junctions and traffic lights and this type of training may be easier to perform on the turbo trainer.

Turbo trainers

The turbo trainer should be set up correctly, bolts tightened and the cycle attached firmly. The attachment for the front forks in particular should be carefully inspected. As you are stationary there is no heat loss through the effect of the wind, and you can become very hot. By using a fan to create wind you can improve heat loss and comfort. Fluid loss through sweating and evaporation is inevitable, so fluid replacement is important even when on the turbo. Clothing should be light and easily removed.

Fartlek

Fartlek is a form of interval training where the intervals are not strictly determined being altered to suit the terrain. There is no specific load, intensity, or recovery period. *Fartlek* is a very natural form of cycle training and we probably all do it subconsciously during long training runs in the countryside. We tend to ride hard up hills, but relatively easier downhill, and use a high gear on long straight stretches of road. This means that we alter the heart rate and physiological loads throughout the training spin. *Fartlek* is usually made up of periods of intense riding followed by rest periods of variable duration, and is really a form of unstructured interval training.

Sprint training

Sprint training improves your absolute speed and is anaerobic. This type of training aims to develop the sheer speed necessary for all road racing. There are many speed training programmes available but they all follow the same general principle. The essential component is a flat out sprint of no more than 200m followed by a period of complete recovery. In practice most coaching manuals suggest that you do repetitions between two fixed points, for example between lampposts etc. The programme may be made up of ladders, pairs, alternate lampposts, and various permutations of short distance work, but must be composed of these short bursts of maximum speed with complete recovery. This type of programme trains essentially fast twitch fibres.

Criterium riders may attempt more specific training where you seek out a circuit and practice sprints out of corners and accelerations on the straight. This follows closely the most important principle of training for any sport: specificity, ie practice the skills of the sport itself.

Sex and training

Sex will not harm your performance in sport. There are many rumours, legends, and clear mistruths in cycling folklore. There is no need for celibacy to improve your sporting performance. Indeed it is not so much the relationship itself that may harm performance as the disco, lack of sleep and effort expended in chasing a partner!

Energy needs

Cycling events may be classified according to the energy pathways. Sprinters require a very fast energy supply to their muscles. These are the ATP-PC and 'fast' intracellular energy sources. The pursuit event requires a fast start and then a sustained high intensity effort. Thus it requires an initial intracellular alactic component, followed by lactic anaerobic component and oxidative carbohydrate metabolism. The endurance event needs a constant energy supply over a longer period, up to four hours at times and so depends on oxidative carbohydrate and fat metabolism with a contribution from calories actually consumed while cycling. Energy produced while cycling in endurance events is produced from oxidation of carbohydrate in glycogen substrate and fatty acid oxidation. Endurance athletes in training have increased their ability to contribute to the energy pool by utilisation of fat metabolism. However fat metabolism depends on low production of lactate, as lactate is a potent inhibitor of fat metabolism. Cyclists train this ability by long slow distance. Fats and carbohydrates contribute to metabolism during endurance exercise, but during more intense work glycogen is the primary fuel. Road racing is a series of intense bursts of activity superimposed on a background of endurance work. Glycogen depletion tends to occur first in the fast twitch glycolytic, followed by the fast twitch oxidative, and then in slow twitch. Glycogen sparing and efficient energy utilisation is fundamental to cycle racing performance.

OVERTRAINING

Our ability to compete in endurance sport is determined to a great degree by the physiological attributes we inherit from our parents. We are born with a potential to perform and unfortunately cannot exceed this potential but we can make the most of it. Genetic potential may be the essential component, but training is the most important determinant of actual performance on the bike. Training aims to develop our genetic potential and translate that potential into tangible performance. There are many essential features of training to maximise performance.

Training must be specific. It must develop the features of fitness that are important in a sport. To be a great distance runner one must train at running, to be a great rower one must concentrate on rowing and to excel in cycling you must train on your bike. However it is not enough simply to cycle. Training must be tailored to improve performance and the fundamental principle of that training is 'overload and recovery'.

Training load

When the body is working with a physiological load, it responds and adapts to cope with that load efficiently. Overload means stressing the body with a load greater than it can cope with easily. This extra loading stimulates improvement. In cycling, the physiological load may be distance and/or speed so increased load means increasing the training distance and/or adding a speed component. If your body is allowed to recover it adapts to cope more easily with this distance and speed, but if you do not increase the load then the body will remain at that initial level of fitness and performance will fail to improve

Important determinants of training effect include not only the intensity and duration of the load but the duration of the recovery. Both are equally important. If the load is excessive or recovery inadequate then the training effect is lost as the body is unable to adapt. If the load and recovery remain inappropriate the body breaks down and not only do we not improve, but our performance is also impaired. It is important to monitor both load and recovery.

A general principle in training is that loading should not be increased by increments greater than 10% per week. This applies to both speed and distance thus it is inappropriate to increase either by more than 10% in any one week.

Recovery means rest or relative rest. Rest allows the body an opportunity to recover from the previous load and prepare for the next load. It means physical and psychological rebuilding and these two features, load and recovery, go hand in hand. Let us look at a typical example: if you complete a very long and fast training ride on a Sunday then you will clearly be very tired on Sunday evening. You may still be tired on Monday, but by Tuesday should be feeling fit and enthusiastic for further training. If the long training session has the desired effect then you will be better able to cope with a similarly long and fast training session in the future. However if you decide next week to cycle twice as far, then you will find you are unable to cope with the increased distance and cannot go as fast. The load is too great, you are unable to cope and lose the training effect. If on the other hand you decided to gradually increase the distance every week then you would soon manage the increased distance at the optimum speed.

Younger or less experienced cyclists often attempt to increase mileage too soon and are unable to recover. Older and more experienced cyclists may fall into the same trap when they try to increase mileage excessively either at the beginning of the season or after injury. Training load must be increased gradually.

If you are pleased with the long training run on Sunday and decide to train hard on Monday, Tuesday and every day the following week you may also run into problems. If your body is inadequately recovered your results on successive days will deteriorate. It is not possible to train hard every day without a drop in performance.

These principles of overload and recovery form the foundation for all training programmes. Training programmes in every sport are based on finding the appropriate load and providing adequate recovery. It is also important to remember that every cyclist is different and a training programme must be tailored to the individual. Training programmes taken from a book should only act as a general guideline and not be read as tablets of stone!

Classic overtraining

Overtraining describes the downward spiral of worsening performance that occurs if we neglect recovery. We are all familiar with the following scenario. A keen and determined rider, who has trained conscientiously, cannot understand his drop in performance. He trains longer and harder but the performance continues to drop and his loss of form meets with increasing depression. Overtraining only seems to occur in the determined and conscientious, but it is often this personality type who fails to see what is happening. Training programmes should be tailored to the individual and gauged to the individual's ability, strengths and weaknesses. However there are many other factors other than the ability and training programme of the cyclist that can influence performance.

Factors totally unrelated may tip the balance between load and recovery. It may not be the training load alone, but the cumulative stress of life that pushes the athlete into overtraining. Other life events, such as exams, personal stress, and work problems are additive so training loads must not be seen in isolation. During exams or other difficult periods training loads should be reduced. The most important psychological determinant of performance is enthusiasm and the keenness to train. If for any reason this enthusiasm is missing performance will be reduced. Performance must be seen in the context of job, lifestyle and workload. The athlete who works hard every day and trains in the evening cannot expect to maintain the same workload as the cyclist who trains for three hours and has the remainder of the day to recover. On the other hand the athlete who has nothing to do all may become bored, disinterested and training become a burden. An athlete's personal situation may in different circumstances be to their advantage or disadvantage.

Other factors may also influence performance. You cannot expect to maintain a suitable training programme without eating an adequate, balanced and sensible diet. A hectic social life of late nights and 'the few beers' will eventually take their toll. While not advocating a monastic lifestyle, these other factors must be taken into consideration. On the other hand, a life of training and racing, early nights and rigorous discipline can also become a life of drudgery. The balance is important and finding the perfect formula, the ideal combination of work, training and play is the key to improving performance.

How to monitor training to prevent overtraining

There are objective and subjective methods of monitoring training and recovery. One of the parameters used to monitor performance and recovery is resting heart rate. Many are aware of pulse rate monitoring in physiological assessment and are aware of the relationship between resting heart rate and fitness. Monitoring morning pulse rate may also act as a guide to general well being. Your pulse rate should be counted first thing in the morning before getting out of bed. Count for a fixed period, for example 10 seconds, and multiply by six to give the pulse rate per minute. Mark this down in a note book. If for any reason there is a rise in the pulse rate of three beats per minute then think seriously about the cause. Are you tired? Have you been training excessively, or is there some other aspect of lifestyle that has altered, affecting performance.

Measuring pulse rate is an excellent method of monitoring recovery after moving to altitude or going across time zones. Overtraining states may be due to chronic dehydration so monitor urine output in terms of colour and total volume. Loss of libido or sex drive is a well-known hazard. Not many athletes report this to their doctor but it is a recognised feature of overtraining!

Depression

Depression in the medical understanding of the word, does not necessarily mean profound sadness, but is a condition that covers many symptoms. These may include a general loss of interest in life, work, family, hobbies and indeed cycling. You will notice that these are also many of the features of overtraining. If during a period of heavy training, the cyclist loses interest in the sport, feels an overwhelming fatigue, or simply cannot face cycling then perhaps they should ask if this could be due to overtraining or staleness. Excessive tiredness or irritability may also reflect an overtraining syndrome. It is interesting to note how many of these symptoms are similar to the clinical features of medical depression.

Treatment

The treatment of overtraining is rest and recovery. Often when the conscientious and determined athlete notes a decreasing performance the natural reaction is to train harder. In an already overtrained athlete this leads to the downward spiral of poor performance, more training, less interest and so on. Monitor the features of overtraining and with unexpected poor performance take care.

In the initial stages this rest and recovery may simply mean a reduction in training load. Psychological rest may be aided by a change in the type of training or a change in terrain. If you regularly go out on your own, then try going out with the club. If your programme includes a lot of interval training then change to a more relaxed aerobic programme. In more severe overtraining syndromes the only option is complete rest. If complete rest is needed then be sure to stick to this rigidly. The temptation to break the rest may be overwhelming and you may go back to training just to check on recovery! You may be tempted to try a training spin and very often the initial tiredness eases as the training spin progresses and towards the end of the session training appears to have returned to normal. You may fool yourself into thinking the slump has ended but if the quality of training and racing remains poor then you really need a prolonged period of rest.

CHAPTER 8

WEIGHT
TRAINING

Weight training and gym work have always been considered an integral part of any cycle training programme. However, as we become more and more aware of the scientific background to training, questions are asked about its relevance to a dedicated cyclist. One benefit may be in maintenance of general fitness and muscle strength, which may deteriorate in the serious rider even if cycling specific fitness is exceptional. As cycle training is very specific, you use few of the other main muscle groups of the body, other than the lower limb so you should do some other additional training, at least to maintain muscle tone and strength, of the other muscle groups.

As if training on the roads was not hazardous enough, weight training brings new dangers! Most cyclists are unaccustomed to weight training and should be aware of the potential for injury. When performing weight training you should learn and use the correct technique and wear a weights belt to support your back. To avoid back injury lift weights off the floor with a straight back, generating the main power using the legs. The knees are flexed and the weight lifted while maintaining a straight back, in this way stresses are transmitted directly along the spinal bones. Indeed this technique should be used for all lifting during the normal course of daily living. Chronic ligamentous low backache is a common problem in cyclists so not only should you take care with bike posture and training but should be very careful when lifting weights.

A weight lifting belt offers some back protection. It enables you to contract your abdominal muscles, increasing intra abdominal pressure which means there is less stress taken directly by the back. Prior to weight training you should do a proper warm up. A typical warm-up routine would include many varied exercises to lightly stress the different muscle groups used in weight training. These exercises should increase muscle temperature and blood flow which improves efficiency and reduces injury. It aids the muscles ability to generate muscle tension and cope with stretch. Your warm up should be at sufficient intensity to increase temperature and blood flow but should not be competitive. A well-planned warm up will use all the various muscle groups used throughout their range of movement.

A standard warm-up routine would begin with a short run to raise heart rate and increase muscle temperature followed by a programme of basic body exercises. A suitable programme would include some or most of the following exercises designed to contract or stretch appropriate muscles, these may include:

- Sit up
- Press up
- Squat jump
- Burpee
- Press up on a chair

- Step up
- Scissors
- Sit up with rotation
- Back extension

The weight training programme itself would most likely include the following exercises:

Power clean

This is one of the foundation exercises in any weight training programme and trains the leg extensors the back extensors and the arm flexors. In this particular exercise it is essential that power be generated off the floor through the legs without using the back.

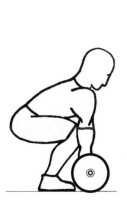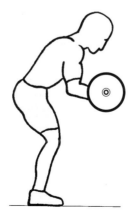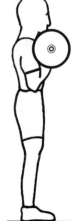

As the bar is accelerated in the initial phase of the lift there should be sufficient momentum for the technically competent athlete to get in under the bar while it is still moving upwards. Proper technique is important. Injuries can occur during the lift if the bottom is not tucked in underneath and the bar is not lifted with a straight back. Poor technique may cause chronic ligamentous back pain. It is important that when lifting, the eyes should be looking forward. The bottom should be tucked in underneath the back and, when using heavy weights, there should be spotters to assist should you be unable to control the bar. During unaccustomed weight training there may be pain in the wrist from flexion and extension as the bar is rotated. Fatigue of these muscles may mean poor control of the bar and can cause injury.

Squats

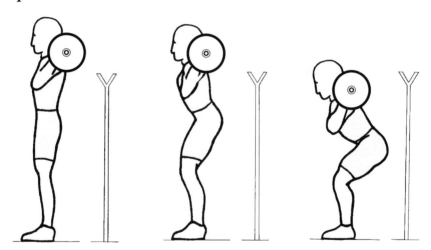

The bar is held across the shoulders behind the neck. The back is held straight and the weight lifted by squatting. This exercise trains primarily the quadriceps muscle group. With heavy weight squats there should be spotters who can catch the bar if you cannot cope with weight that is too heavy. A squat should not be too deep. The depth of the squat may be gauged by the angle of the thigh. The femur, or thigh bone, should not be at an angle more than horizontal to the floor. Squat exercises that are too deep may cause knee problems, a hazard that we have already identified as a feature of cycling.

Sit ups

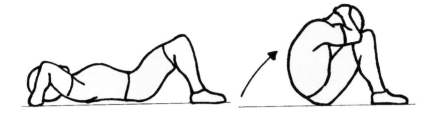

Sit ups may be of particular benefit to the cyclist who often has poor posture with poor abdominal musculature. Keep the knees flexed, which ensures that only the abdominal muscles are used. With straight legs it is possible to use the hip flexors, the psoas and iliacus muscles, to aid the abdominal muscles but flexing the knees ensures abdominal muscles alone are used. It is important to emphasis the importance of the abdominal muscle development in cyclists where poor musculature may be a major factor in the poor posture leading to low back pain.

Bench press

Lie on a stable, well-supported bench. The weight should be held in a rack, and with heavy weights, you should always have spotters. In this exercise you grasp the weight and lower and raise the weight to the chest by flexion of the elbow and the shoulder. You will need spotters if using heavy weights, so you do not get trapped by a heavy bar that you cannot lift off the chest.

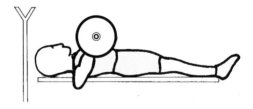

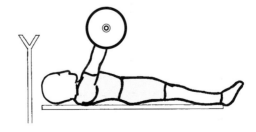

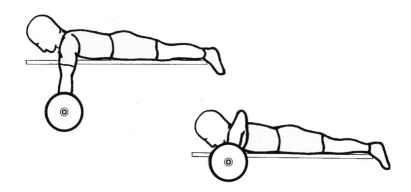

High pull

Lie on a raised, stable, and well-supported bench, with the bar supported on a ledge. You then lift the weight off the ledge and lower and raise the weight using the arm and shoulder flexor muscles. There is less risk of injury with this exercise as you can drop the weight if necessary. Unilateral high pulls should be avoided by cyclists because they do not have appropriate muscle development and may be injured.

Footwear

You should wear correct footwear in the gym. Running shoes are not ideal as your training shoe should be stable and not have a large heel counter. It should have a moderate heel wedge however so that the Achilles tendon is not stretched.

Other sports

Cyclists play football, basketball, and other sports during the winter and off-season, but an occasional game is sure to leave you with multiple aches and pains! Fitness is specific and there is little cross over to other sports. In particular, your muscles are accustomed to the smooth silky non-traumatic movements on the bike. They are not trained to cope with jarring movements on a hard surface or constant changes in direction and speed. Playing a contact sport will incur the same aches and pains as a novice. Injuries can occur in these sports and if as a cyclist, you are not accustomed to playing, you may have neither the skill nor the muscle development to play these sports safely. Generally, cyclists may have poor spatial awareness and lack the ability to judge speed and other player's movements. You do not have the same muscle balance or the proprioceptive joint awareness. If the games are competitive games the cyclist, who is a natural competitor, will compete and probably take risks. It therefore follows that a cyclist who plays contact sports occasionally is more likely to become injured than those sports people who play contact sports regularly.

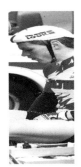

CHAPTER 9

RACING

A ny rider, independent of their ability, should try to maximise their talent. This means trying to achieve the very best from their physiological potential. We cannot all be champions or winners of the Tour, but true success in sport is to achieve the best results possible. Riders should have a goal: this may be to win a national classic, become an international, win a yellow jersey or perhaps most of us should have more modest objectives such as to finish a stage race, or to finish first in a third catagory open race. A modest goal attained may reflect an achievement as great as being world champion, depending on your ability. Attaining your goals requires a lot of preparation.

PRE-RACE TRAINING

During the winter you should plan a schedule for weeks or months ahead and build into it a programme of cycling, running and/or weight training. The winter provides an opportunity to catch up on all those jobs at home or at work, and to relax and to recover from last year's racing. Make the most of it because these opportunities may not be available in the season ahead.

Although your training hours need not necessarily be long, your training programme should be structured and monitored from week to week as the winter progresses. As the racing season approaches more time will be spent on the bike and the priority will be cycle training during daylight. Weekends are the most important phase of training when you may do longer hours. It is important that this training is planned and structured but also enjoyable and stimulating.

During this time of the year you may get most value from the club run as it allows you to maintain an aerobic base. Although there may be little gain in training effect, these long club rides prevent loss of aerobic fitness. It also means that you can enjoy the camaraderie and companionship of colleagues on the bike without the stress of racing. Be careful however that the training does not degenerate into a race as this serves no purpose to any athlete in the winter time. There are no prizes in the winter races!

Your lifestyle should be directed towards getting the most benefit from training. Any athlete should avoid too many late nights, excess alcohol, and look after their body well, which means in any sport eating a good balanced sensible diet and modifying all aspects of lifestyle to improve performance. This is basic common sense. There are no hard and fast rules on drinking alcohol, as each individual's ability to cope with alcohol depends on their size and liver metabolism, but alcohol intake should be limited so it does not affect the ability to perform in training. You need not set a curfew for bed time but, suffice to say, you should maintain some regularity of lifestyle and ensure adequate rest. If you are a serious cyclist you will spend considerable time training and racing; undoubtably you will make sacrifices in many other aspects of life so it is only reasonable to ensure that the sacrifices made are worthwhile.

EQUIPMENT

The cycle industry is big business and considerable emphasis is placed on marketing new equipment. There are however few genuine revolutionary new ideas in cycle equipment and equipment alone will not make the bike go faster. The engine is more important.

Caring for the equipment should not be an end in itself. A bike will not go faster because it is painted more prettily or shines brighter in the sun, but a poorly maintained bike may not only slow you down but may cost the race through its failure.

BEFORE THE RACE

Preparation for a race requires common sense. It demands some thought to plan travel arrangements, meals, rest, accommodation etc. You should plan to arrive at the start long before the race. Sitting in a car continuously for three to four hours is not the best preparation for any athletic event so stop along the way, rest, stretch the legs and perhaps limber up with a short jog. Arrive well before the event and stay loose, relaxed and ready to go. Have clean equipment and clean racing kit. Clean gear will not of course make you go any faster but it is good for morale and gives a psychological lift.

Warm up before the event. A warm up has a number of benefits, not just physiological. It allows you to check your equipment and make any necessary adjustments. It is important to warm down after the race, do some general stretching and change clothes to keep warm.

Physical performance and psychological readiness are very closely interwoven. It is not necessary to psyche yourself up but those who have prepared sensibly, looked after themselves and looked after their equipment will have a better belief in themselves and in their ability.

Preparation is the key. A race will not be won in the 24 hours beforehand but it can very easily be lost. Beware of great new ideas to aid performance. Very often what we hear in the media or what makes good TV are the more unusual features of athletic performance and it would be a mistake to think that everything one sees or hears is ideal. You can appreciate that if a rider's diet in the Tour of France was two fried egg sandwiches and a bottle of Chianti, this would make much more exciting news than a sensible carbohydrate diet with proper fluid replacement. What we read may make good news but may not make good sense. Genuine improvements come by evolution and occur slowly. Greet any new wonderful idea with a healthy scepticism as there are few exceptions to hard work and good preparation.

STAGE RACING

The stage race is unique to cycling with its daily sequence of high-intensity, long duration competition causing considerable physical and psychological stress. You must prepare well, take care of yourself during the event, and ensure complete recovery. Here are some medical physiological and nutritional issues to consider in your preparations:

DIET

During training your intake should contain all the natural nutrients of a normal balanced diet. While this is relatively easy to achieve in the normal pattern of daily living, during a stage race the entire pattern of the day is altered. Your calorie needs are considerably increased, and there is little control over diet and meal times. Whereas during normal daily training the emphasis is on maintaining a well-balanced diet, the emphasis during a stage race must be on maintaining sufficient calorie intake to fuel your muscles for each successive stage. Carbohydrate is the most appropriate food for replacement of energy need. Thus, during a major multi-day stage race you should consume a high carbohydrate diet with pasta, potato, bread and vegetables being the major constituents. Increased protein is not necessary so the quality or quantity of meat is relatively unimportant. Intake of fats should always be minimal.

The dietary preparation for the stage begins with breakfast, which should of course be composed mainly of carbohydrate. An appropriate breakfast may contain cereal, bread with jam or honey and plenty of fluid. A traditional fried breakfast would be a most inappropriate start to a cyclist's day. Not only is the fat and protein content a slow and inefficient form of fuel, but also the fat content of fried food slows down stomach emptying. Some cyclists prefer rice or pasta for breakfast during a stage race, and this is nutritionally correct, if perhaps a little difficult to face first thing in the morning! The major morning meal should be eaten about three hours before the start of the stage and any later food before the start should be a light snack, for example, tea and toast or a cereal bar with plenty of fluids. During the stage the two important dietary considerations are calorie and fluid intake. It is important to remember that you are not only racing today but preparing for tomorrow, so during each stage you should maintain hydration and calorie intake. If you become dehydrated or calorie depleted during today's stage it is increasingly difficult to replace fluid and fuel before the following day's stage. During the stage you should drink freely if possible, and should be sipping water constantly throughout the evening.

It is important to eat adequate correct food. Scientists may point out that the ideal calorie replacement during a stage is a glucose or glucose polymer solution without the need for solid food. However a major race is not the right time to experiment and unless one has tried this form of nutrition before, it is best to eat and drink what you are used to from previous races. If you eat during the stage carbohydrate in the form of sugar bars, fruit, and cake is much more suitable than high fat snacks containing chocolate.

The most important consideration regarding food in stage racing is to maintain adequate fuel supply to the muscles. The period immediately after the completion of a stage, and up to one hour after is an important time for recovery of muscle fuel stores. Muscles are especially hungry for glycogen and muscle enzymes are at their most efficient. If possible you should have a carbohydrate snack immediately after the stage, ie a cup of tea and sandwich or biscuit. Do not wait until the evening meal which may not be for one or two hours after the stage as the period immediately after the stage is critical. The evening meal may be a traditional meal, but with particular emphasis on carbohydrate, where potatoes and vegetables are of more nutritional importance than meat or high fat desert. Remember that the cyclist who loses weight during a stage race has clearly not been eating adequate food to match fuel needs.

ILLNESS AND INJURY

The increased mileage and intensity of a stage race may cause old injuries to recur. The increased workload of a major national tour will find any weakness. You should not start a major stage race carrying an injury. The injury will certainly not ease and the intensity and physical stress on the body during a major stage race will magnify the effects of any injury. Tendinitis or muscle injury may be treated during the race, but classic cyclist's knee pain will always get worse. With severe knee pain you should abandon the race because if you continue in a race of this intensity, the injury may deteriorate sufficiently to cost you the remainder of the season.

Coughs, colds and sore throats may occur during the race just as at any other time of the year. Mild respiratory symptoms may not be significant but any infection causing a temperature or muscle aches and pains is a warning not to continue. You will not do yourself justice in the race, and it may be positively harmful to your health. Any illness causing a temperature or muscle ache may also cause inflammation of the heart muscle and by riding hard you may damage your heart. It may be useful to bring along some simple medicines: aspirin or paracetamol, throat lozenges for a dry and irritated throat, Elastoplast, Vaseline and sunscreen should be in everyone's bag. If you use an asthma inhaler, even if only occasionally, be sure to bring it with you. There may be medical facilities at the race but it will help if you bring along your own dressings etc in case of a fall. For hay fever, antihistamines are permitted and some nasal sprays but remember that there is drug testing on most major stage races so be careful that you do not inadvertently take a banned medication. If in doubt speak to the race doctor.

When you start a stage race if all your preparation has been completed then nothing further, in theory, can be done to improve your performance. Only one cyclist can win each race, but that does not mean that only one has been successful. There may be as much satisfaction in finishing in the bunch as there is in winning. It may be just as hard for a novice cyclist to hang on the back of the pack as it is for the elite athlete at the front to win. Remember that the cyclist who wins the regional event easily is the same one who struggles at the back of the international event. There is only one world champion! It is important to enjoy your success. Part of fulfilment in cycling is the achievement of your potential in the sport.

CHAPTER 10

TRAINING YOUR MIND

Psychology plays a major part in the preparation and performance of many sports. Motivation and ambition must be carefully nurtured and focused. It is not enough to have raw hunger, you must be able to control and guide training through the inevitably long period of preparation. As the competition period approaches you must be able to control the anxiety and tension associated with the event in order to gain the best in performance.

Training period

For most sports there is a long and sustained period of preparation over months and years and peak performance is only achieved after investment of considerable time and effort. Champions may be lucky to have been born with natural talent but this talent will only produce results if nurtured through training. Only those with an almost obsessive ambition are prepared to invest the time and effort required to succeed and all champions have this obsessive ambition. Athletes, in any sport, only succeed if they have driving ambition but direction, control and channelling of this ambition is an important aspect of preparation for any sport.

The committed individual is more likely to overtrain, so control often means holding back and redirection of training effort. Excessive training can bring burnout, and misdirected training may mean that you either produce your best performances in training or at the wrong time in the racing season. Most athletes need some form of objective advice, hence the importance of a coach who may advise on level and intensity of training and help to produce the best performance at the optimum time.

Modern coaching theory has structured this type of controlled training into periodic cycles. There are many sophisticated training schedules emphasising mini cycles, macrocycles, peaks and recovery. However the common feature of all programmes is a period of intense effort combined with a period of relative rest.

The race

In many sports the period of competition is short and intense with all the activity happening in a short concentrated timespan, for example in sprint racing. Road racing cyclists are accustomed to a very different timespan. Psychological preparation therefore demands a different protocol. There are peaks of concentration and intense physical effort superimposed on a constant high load. These are periods in the race during which there is intense activity with attacks, counterattacks and blocking and you must be especially alert during these periods of activity.

A critical time is just after the start when you must be alert to what is happening in the bunch, to maintain position and be aware of your team-mates position. This period of excitement occurs before the race settles down, with constant movement, ebb and flow and where the slightest loss of concentration may mean you miss a crucial break or perhaps cause a crash. Once the race has settled you must be aware of what is happening and be prepared to cope with any eventuality.

As the race progresses you may tire, but when the going gets hard this requires mental toughness, guts and determination. In the winning break the athletes are usually all of high quality, but the winner is the one who can play the game of psychological poker to the greatest advantage. It also requires shrewd tactical awareness to know the important breaks and spot the significant moves. Being 'over psyched' or over motivated may also handicap the cyclist as an aggressive ride may not always gain results in the end. The cyclist who chases every move and leads out all his competitors will be beaten by one who, though less physically capable, has managed to conserve energy until it is needed and uses it with devastating effect.

Track racing requires a more specialised form of psychological preparation. These are shorter more intense events which require more focused preparation. The event, whether a track sprint or a pursuit demands total concentration. You must have a blinkered yet highly alert mind and this intense focused concentration may be trained.

Psychological preparation

It is difficult to create big event conditions and atmosphere in training so riders may learn psychological exercises to prepare for the big event. One technique is visualisation or mental rehearsal.

Anxiety and tension are a natural response to the stress of competition. They are the signs of the bodies readiness for competition and are thus essential for peak performance. Mental rehearsal and visualisation are a means of coming to terms with this anxiety and harnessing them to best effect.

The technique is as follows. You try to imagine the event, and all its aspects including every possible scenario so that when it comes to the actual moment you are already mentally prepared for every possibility. You have seen in your mind's eye all the razzmatazz and distractions of the event and are familiar with them. By the time of actual competition you can then concentrate fully and focus on the event closing out all other stimuli.

Over excitedness, called overarousal, can also inhibit performance. There are folk descriptions of this phenomenon with which we are familiar: 'the choker' 'over the top' 'always cracks at the big one'. It is possible to develop techniques to master pre-event nerves and overstress and so get the best out of yourself when it counts most. Autogenic relaxation is such a technique where you learn to be aware of all the symptoms of anxiety and their effect prior to the event, so that you know that the symptoms of dry mouth, 'butterflies in the tummy', the feeling of fatigue, exhaustion, and heart thumping are all natural and normal features of preparation. These are the somatic symptoms of anxiety and by focusing on these symptoms you may make a conscious effort to control them.

It is important to realise that these symptoms are of positive value, that they are indeed essential for good performance, and bearing this in mind you can appreciate that even though you may feel wretched in the minutes or hours before competition, these symptoms are the body's way of preparing for competition, and are indeed of great benefit. Understanding and learning to cope with the almost overwhelming waves of anxiety helps produce your best performance on the day.

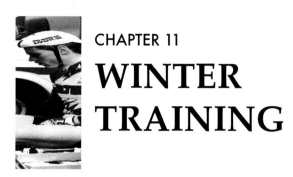

CHAPTER 11

WINTER TRAINING

The cool September breezes and the early darkening evenings herald the end of the domestic cycling season, but the end of the season does not mean the end of training. While it may be a well earned opportunity to rest and recover from the rigours of the past season, it is important to remain in shape.

Your fitness can deteriorate quite quickly if neglected. While the winter months mean the end of racing for this year they are also the preparation period for the season to come. Rest means relative rest, so while winter means that you may reduce the volume and intensity of training, it is also an opportunity to vary the type of training and develop aspects of fitness that you may have omitted during racing.

Fitness has two components: central fitness or cardiovascular fitness, and peripheral fitness or local muscle endurance. Cardiovascular fitness means training the heart and improving its efficiency as a pump. Local muscle endurance training means improving the efficiency of the muscles and their ability to use the fuel supplied in the bloodstream (ie oxygen and energy substrate). Any form of endurance sport that raises heart rate to a training threshold will have a cardiovascular training effect, but local muscle fitness is very specific and is best gained by using those muscles at the speed and in the sequence used when cycling.

TYPES OF TRAINING

Cycling is essentially an aerobic sport so it is important that you maintain an endurance or aerobic base during winter. Aerobic exercise is sustained exercise at an intensity that makes you breathe quite hard. There are a number of ways of achieving this type of training. Some cyclists run, some swim, and recently many have begun to use mountain bikes. Cyclo cross has always been a traditional means of maintaining aerobic fitness during the winter and more recently some continue to use the road bike. Remembering the principle of specificity of fitness there is no doubt that in purely physiological terms the best training for cycling is cycling! After a hard season however, most cyclists are mentally as well as physically tired. It is most important to start the new season mentally refreshed and enthusiastic. It is even more important to be just as enthusiastic in mid season, so although in physiological terms it may be more appropriate to continue to cycle, psychologically it may be prudent to find an alternative type of training to give yourself a proper break.

Swimming

Swimming offers a safe alternative. You are unlikely to become injured in the pool and it provides an opportunity for aerobic sport in a pleasant warm environment. On the other hand, many cyclists are usually not good swimmers and in order to gain aerobic benefits you must have a reasonable level of technical competence. Continuous swimming of 20 to 40 minutes duration offers good cardiovascular or aerobic workout.

There are some medical conditions associated with swimming. Swimmer's ear is a chronic skin inflammation of the ear canal which occurs because the ears become wet and macerated. The inside of the ear canal should be dried gently with a soft towel as this skin is delicate and sensitive. Rough cleansing can break down the skin surface which may become inflamed and infected.

Swimmer's shoulder is a chronic overuse injury of the shoulder due to impingement of muscles of the shoulder. The shoulder muscles called the rotator cuff may be compressed under the bone arch and ligaments of the shoulder when the swimmer draws the arm above the head during the crawl and butterfly stroke. Breast stroker's knee is a chronic medial ligament strain which occurs through stretching in the breast stroke. Conjunctivitis is inflammation of the white of the eye and may be related to chlorine and other preparations used to keep pools clean. If you intend to swim often you should use goggles.

Running

Running is an effective form of aerobic exercise for the cyclist. It is convenient and mimics more closely the cardiovascular load of cycling. Injury is a problem for those unaccustomed to running which includes most cyclists! A suitable training target for maintenance of aerobic fitness is about 40 to 60 minutes of continuous running, but you will not be able to go directly into this type of training after the cycling season. Your legs are accustomed to smooth continuous rotatory movements and are ill prepared for the jarring trauma of running. Start off gently and use good sensible well-cushioned shoes designed specifically for running. The top of the range 8oz racer is not for you as you need support and cushioning. Try to run on grass if at all possible. Cycling traditionalists would throw their hands up in horror at the idea of cyclists running as an integral part of their training. Triathletes have introduced many new ideas and training methods and the inclusion of running is now quite acceptable. Running can enhance winter training, but it is not the complete answer, and you should be aware of the potential for new injuries.

Although cycling and running use similar muscles (the quadriceps at the front of the thigh, hamstring at the back and the soleus and gastrocnemius muscles which make up the calf) the type of muscle contraction is quite different. Cycling is non-weight bearing with a constant smooth, and sustained action. In contrast, with each running step the heel strikes the ground at a force of up to 10 times the body's weight. With each stride the muscle contracts and is sharply stretched at the same time. The impact of each stride not only jars the bones but also stretches the soft tissues, muscles and tendons which causes micro-trauma (muscle damage at cellular level). This may be a factor in the pain and stiffness that occur after unaccustomed exercise.

However, running does offer a good cardiovascular workout, in a concentrated time, without the hazards of cycling in the dark. Running tends to raise body temperature quickly and since speeds are slower than cycling, there is less wind-cooling effect so runners can remain warm and comfortable in conditions that would require Arctic style protection on the bike. Heart rate increases almost immediately when running, and can be maintained fairly easily. Achieving the equivalent cardiovascular load on the bike takes around three times as long. Although cyclists are usually very fit endurance athletes, you may be surprised to discover that you are unable to cope with a 20 minute, low intensity run. Running should be introduced gradually as part of training. Be patient and allow sufficient rest days to let muscles recover fully.

Running training programmes are very similar in structure to the normal cycling training schedule programme, with long slow distance, *fartlek*, intervals, sprints, etc. Aim to run two to three times a week for periods of 30–50 minutes. *Fartlek*, or speed play is like an unstructured interval and may be introduced once a week. Intervals provide an extra cardiovascular load, but cyclists should probably keep away from running speed work on the track. Increasing the intensity and duration of running too quickly after the cycling season can cause injury and a common overuse injury is stress fractures. Cycling bones are not accustomed to impact stress and may develop tiny fractures – similar to the metal fatigue that may occur in aircraft wings. This type of injury often affects the shins, where it is called shin splints.

A typical story is the pain which occurs when running and becomes more severe as the run progresses. As it becomes worse pain may also occur at rest or at night. The treatment is rest but prevention is always preferable to cure, and stress fractures may be prevented by increasing running mileage gradually. Try to train on a forgiving surface: grass is ideal, and asphalt is less stressful than concrete. Sand can be a high impact surface, particularly close to the water's edge where it is packed hard. The Achilles tendon also undergoes considerable stretch and stress while running and is susceptible to overuse injury. Abnormalities in running gait, common in cyclists, and inappropriate shoes may aggravate the problem. Running can be safe and convenient, and offers a chance to maintain cardiovascular fitness, but try to maintain weekend training rides, even in the off-season.

Mountain biking

Mountain biking brings a new and exciting dimension to winter bike training. It has all the benefits of aerobic training and uses muscles groups appropriate to road racing. It also offers the pleasure of spending those fine crisp winter weekends in the heather and bracken of our beautiful countryside. There must be some catch! Your mountain bike may be set up differently to your road bike and may not have toe clips and without toe clips your pedalling technique is different. Mountain bikers usually train on mountains, and excess climbing can cause knee pain. Mountain biking is good winter cycle training but is not a perfect substitute for road biking. Mountain biking tends to be a lower cadence than road biking and the use of flat pedals without clips or straps means that you may lose the silky smooth rotatory muscle action that develops from spinning on the road, but mountain biking is still useful sport for winter training. Remember also that training with your club mates and friends can often deteriorate into a racing session. You do not want to become racing stale. You want your best races during the racing season, there are no prizes on a wet Saturday in November!

Winter weight training and gym work

The cyclist is really a cardiovascular and local muscle endurance machine. The absolute resistance on the pedal during cycling is not great, so there is no great need for pure strength training. The emphasis in gym work should not be on weight or strength training, but more on the cardiovascular component of circuit training. Resistance is not important but speed and continuous movement are fundamental. Look however at the posture of the racing cyclist. Through long periods of cycling the lower limbs are well developed, but there is relative inactivity of the upper body and abdominal muscles. A winter programme of training using body weight exercises and abdominal strengthening helps to prevent the muscle imbalance that can contribute to future injury. With weight training the emphasis should be more on the 'training' than the weight, and winter training should be general training of all muscle groups rather than just the legs.

Pure weight training is not of specific advantage in cycling but speed endurance is. Weight training should thus be directed towards improving local muscle endurance using low weights and high repetitions. Circuits of 10–12 exercises of 10–30 repetitions using different muscle groups continuously for 20–30 minutes provide a very useful form of training. Naturally, this must be done at a sufficient speed and intensity to raise the heart rate to a training threshold. In this way, circuit training may be of benefit to both the cardiovascular and local muscle endurance components of training. As in all weight training programmes it is especially important to warm up, warm down and include stretching routines.

Triathlon

Cyclists often attempt triathlons for variety or as part of their training and not just in winter. Cross training reduces the potential for overuse injury because of the variety of training for each sport.

On the other hand the triathletes will be exposed to all the risks and injury of each individual sport. Training is specific and not necessarily transferable so although cardiovascular fitness is common to all endurance sports, the physiological benefits from running or swimming are not completely transferable to cycling.

Cyclists should be aware of the hazards of sea swimming, in particular the cold and risk of hypothermia. Wet suits are permitted in most triathlons depending on water temperature and it helps to get used to swimming in cold water in lakes or the sea. Modern wet suits are a considerable development from early wet suits used in skin diving. They are more flexible and allow greater range of movement while maintaining body temperature and providing some buoyancy. Wet suits also improve the swimming times of triathletes. Hard shell helmets are compulsory and indeed the triathlon governing body gave the lead by being first to make hard shells mandatory.

Skiing

Downhill skiing is exciting, colourful, dramatic and trendy. Surely this is the ideal sport for the image-conscious cyclist! After all we often see photographs of the professional teams on the ski slopes at the pre-season get together. But how will it benefit the cyclist in training? Physiologically speaking, very little. There is little cardiovascular load in downhill skiing. There is muscular contraction, predominantly isometric, in the legs, but there is little isotonic muscle activity unless the athlete is a very skilled skier and participating in slalom type activity. Skiing is great fun, great for mental relaxation, but of minimal fitness benefit.

Cross-country skiing

Let the poseurs go downhill. Real athletes go *langlauf!* Cross-country skiing is the ultimate endurance sport and some of the highest oxygen uptake values have been measured in cross-country skiers. There is sustained muscle contraction in the legs using quads, hamstrings and calves and cross-country skiing is atraumatic. It involves local muscle endurance training, as in cycling, but without the constant repetitive trauma of running. The arms are used for propulsion thereby training the shoulder girdle. The cardiovascular training benefit goes without saying so cross-country skiing is an ideal form of endurance training for the cyclist.

Rowing

Contrary to most people's perceptions, rowing is a high intensity endurance sport which stresses most large muscle groups but especially the legs. High level training demands a maximum leg contraction at the start of the stroke, predominantly the quadriceps muscle group. The large muscle groups of the back continue the drive phase and the oar is drawn up to the body at the finish of the stroke using the arms and the shoulders. The rowing cadence is 24–36 strokes per minute, which is less than running or cycling but the leg extension is similar to cycling.

One major problem for cyclists wishing to row is that they must be proficient to achieve a training effect. Rowers can often transfer to cycling without difficulty as cardiovascular fitness is transferable and cycling may already be part of their training programme, but cyclists need to develop rowing skills before gaining training benefits. In addition, most cyclists have poorly developed upper body musculature which puts them at a distinct disadvantage in rowing.

Rowing clubs are unlikely to encourage cyclists to join, fearing that they learn to row in a crew and then abandon it in the summer when the racing season runs concurrently with the regatta season.

Aerobics

Aerobics may mean different things to different people. If aerobics means a continuous intense workout, then it may promote cardiovascular endurance, but a gentle stretch routine in a leotard will hardly raise the heart rate to any useful degree.

Diverse aerobic exercises which involve a variety of muscle movements will improve flexibility. This is of particular benefit to the cyclist whose sport-specific training plan does not allow general leisure activities and stretching. Greater flexibility will mean improved back mobility for cycling but the muscle action and nature of aerobics are unlikely to offer a specific training effect.

There is no valid substitute for sustained intensive and extensive training on the bike. During the winter and off-season you may experiment with other forms of training to provide mental relief and yet maintain some training effect. Each sport offers different potential benefits, but remember that fitness is so specific that training in a sport simply makes you better at that sport. When you are standing in the line-up before the 'off' the commissaires don't give you a head start because you can ski or row. It is a fundamental principle of all sport, endurance sport in particular, that training is specific. The best form of training for a sport is to do it! Cross training may provide a welcome break while maintaining some components of fitness but the most effective form of cycle training is on the bike.

There is a fine line between load and overload, training and overtraining, adaptation and overuse injury in intense training for endurance sport. For the endurance athlete overuse injuries are the most common form of injury but overuse injury can be reduced by varying the training, practising alternative and cross-training.

Winter training should be fun and enjoyable and offer the opportunity to add flexibility to training. It should also be safe and, bearing in mind that the cyclist is unaccustomed to different forms of training, should be approached with care and respect.

WINTER CLOTHING

Training during winter may be cold, wet, miserable and dangerous. Correct clothing is important to ensure you stay warm, yet remain comfortable and visible in the dark winter afternoons. Non cyclists wonder at the unusual clothing that streetwise cyclists wear on winter training runs: the tights, bibshorts, overshoes, thermal jackets, capes and gloves. This clothing was not discovered overnight but evolved over many years as cyclists experimented and found the most appropriate clothing by trial and error.

Over the years riders have found that many thin layers retain heat better than large bulky clothing. Cyclists usually wear an undershirt often with two or more jerseys and even an old sweater over the undervest. Cotton vests tend to become soaked with sweat and you may become cold if the speed drops or you become tired. Undershirts are available in modern synthetic materials which wick the sweat away from the skin and may be more suitable. However during very hot weather some nylon and synthetic materials do not breathe, and although the undershirt does not become sodden in sweat, it also fails to help heat dissipation, contributing to overheating.

The dimensions of the cycling jersey are determined by the rules of cycle racing. It is important in winter to keep warm and in summer to keep cool so the fabric is all important. Cycling jerseys tend to be manufactured with heat retention in mind. Traditional knitted woollen jerseys provided heat insulation yet did not become sodden when sweating excessively. The more modern jerseys, with synthetic fibres provide improved heat retention yet are not as bulky. The traditional winter top is knitted wool with waterproof panels at the front and on the shoulders. This gives some protection against wind and rain yet allows the clothes to breathe. A fully covered waterproof top does not allow sweat loss so there is condensation on the inside of the waterproof and undergarments become very wet with sweat. More modern thermal tops are extremely effective at heat retention yet allow the fabric to breathe. They are recommended.

The enthusiastic winter cyclist should wear tights, either the traditional woollen tights or thermal leggings. Bib tights offer the added comfort of the higher waist and a warmer back. In addition, the absence of waist elastic helps prevent sweat accumulation at the midriff. Overshoes help prevent cold feet, despite the leg muscles being continuously active, the feet remain relatively static and may become extremely cold even frost-bitten. You should always wear gloves or mittens and thermal gloves are a tremendous advance. Cyclists should always carry a cape, not only to protect against the rain, but it is essential to wear a cape when stopping to fix a puncture or repair a mechanical problem. The cold bitter winter wind quickly changes the warm glow of winter training to shivering numbness. Some find it useful to carry a flask of hot tea or coffee and it is important to eat plenty. Always carry change for the telephone, food, or even the bus!

It also makes sense to wear bright colours that are easily visible in the dark days and early dusk of winter. It seems obvious, but when cycling at night your lights should be working and bright and luminous vests and belts are available which improve the visibility and profile of the cyclist in motorists' eyes.

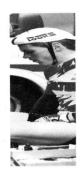

CHAPTER 12

YOUR INTAKE

NUTRITION

Much has been written about nutrition in cycling. The correct diet is central to performance in endurance sport; in fact a careless diet may harm it. Many cyclists are especially interested in diet in an effort to improve their performance. There are many differing thoughts and theories among the cycling community on the appropriate food and fluid intake and while some of it is true, some bears very little, if any, relationship to the accepted principles of optimum nutrition. There are no hard and fast rules about diet and there are no magic formulas for success in sport. There is no one particular food that will make the difference between finishing in the bunch and consistent victories. We can almost all recognise a balanced diet and it is important to use the knowledge that we possess.

There are some basic principles of nutrition that apply in all endurance sports, running, swimming, cycling etc, but grass roots cycling is greatly influenced by what happens among the professionals. Professional cycling differs greatly from amateur cycling, and there are aspects of life on the professional circuit that make it difficult to get an adequate diet. Professionals have a very different lifestyle, spending seven hours on the bike day after day, and so organising a nutritionally balanced diet with traditional meals is difficult. This means that a racer's intake can be quite unorthodox with a need for special supplements and additives. Unfortunately many amateurs believe that these supplements are essential for their own top performance, forgetting that professionals eat this abnormal diet from necessity rather than choice. Naturally, manufacturers and marketing people are slow to point this out and hype the value of vitamins, energy bars and similar products. Very few top amateurs have a lifestyle similar to the professionals, and for most of us, it is not difficult to arrange a healthy balanced diet spread over three meals per day. Rather than look for supplements we should concentrate more on our normal daily diet to ensure that it contains the correct proportions of all nutrients. The average amateur cyclist has little need for vitamin supplements, additives and vitamin injections.

Let us highlight a number of important features of the optimum diet in four key areas:

- the normal training diet
- the pre-race diet
- nutrition during racing
- special dietary needs when stage racing.

Normal training diet

Fats, carbohydrates, and proteins are the building blocks of a normal diet. Most of us are aware of what constitutes the correct diet through widespread health education, but we may find it difficult to put our knowledge into practice. In Europe we generally consume too much fat in our diet ie chocolate, butter, cakes, biscuits, and the first dietary modification should be simply to switch to all those foods we know are good for us, such as fruit, vegetables etc. If you are living at home, eating the normal family diet and enjoying home cooking, it is relatively easy to maintain a good diet. But if you are a student or working full time and trying to fit training time into an already full day, it may be difficult to find the time to buy, prepare, and cook the correct foods. There will be the temptation to eat convenience foods which upset the normal balance of the correct diet. Diet sheets are often published in sports magazines and are usually available from your local sports nutritionist, but while there are many diet sheets and formal guidelines available, most of us do in fact know what we should be eating.

Pre-race food

When you slip your foot into the pedal at the start of a race your fuel tanks should be full and you should be well hydrated. It is impossible to fill those fuel tanks sufficiently in the last five minutes before the race by guzzling large quantities of tea, biscuits rice puddings etc. Those fuel tanks should have been filled in the days prior to the race by reducing training and increasing carbohydrate intake. It is important to taper, or reduce training mileage and intensity, before a major race not only to rest your muscles but also to build up fuel reserves depleted by heavy training. During this preparation period you should eat large quantities of carbohydrate as these are the most efficient food to help muscle to replenish its glycogen stores, the muscle energy source. Eating carbohydrate is similar to filling your car with high octane fuel while protein and fat are like crude oil that the body must refine before use as fuel for racing. Carbohydrates include bread, potatoes, pasta, and vegetables so clearly the correct food need not be expensive.

Glycogen is the muscle energy source. Glycogen enables the body to perform for an extended period and it is essential that these glycogen stores be full prior to endurance events. After each hard training session or race your energy stores are reduced so your diet should aim to replenish them. Glycogen stores must be restored in the 48–72 hours prior to an event, and this is achieved most effectively with a high carbohydrate diet. A typical high carbohydrate diet would contain 60–70% of caloric intake as carbohydrate. Glycogen stores usually contain enough energy for about two hours of intense endurance activity. It has been found that the time taken to exhaust muscles in exercise is closely related to glycogen storage state. Well-trained endurance athletes may eke out their glycogen store to last a little longer as endurance training helps the body to modify its energy needs by using some fat as an energy source. This is known as the glycogen sparing effect of lipid metabolism.

Cyclists often eat a carbohydrate snack prior to a race. Nutritionists may not always agree with this as traditional teaching suggests that high glucose content food prior to an event stimulates an insulin surge which will harm performance. Cyclists have never found this in practice and indeed recent experimental work from Holland also demonstrated that glucose ingestion, even prior to activity, does in fact have a glycogen sparing action. This research suggests that an immediate pre-race snack may be of benefit in helping the body utilise its fuel stores economically during the race. While in many other sports it would be unwise to have a meal or snack immediately before competition, it appears that because of the duration of most cycle races it may be of benefit. In addition, because body weight is supported, cyclists may eat without the usual ill effects of exercising with food in the stomach.

On the morning of the race, you should begin with a light but high carbohydrate breakfast, in practice this means cereal, bread and jam with little butter or a low fat spread. Stay away from fatty foods and fries. Fatty foods are a poor fuel and slow down stomach emptying. You should drink plenty of fluid to ensure adequate hydration and the best fluid is water.

Nutrition during racing

It is important, in events which last longer than two hours, to maintain some caloric intake during the event and most medical opinion favours liquid energy replacement. Fred Bruens, a well-known Dutch scientist with a special expertise in cycling nutrition, performed a huge research project in which he simulated the nutritional needs of a rider in the Tour de France. From this work he suggests that optimal calorie intake is through glucose and glucose polymer drinks. He also emphasised the need for fluid intake during sustained exercise for maintenance of heat regulation. In multi-stage events he found that the ability of cyclists to balance their caloric intake to their workload requirements was reflected in their racing results. Bruens' work validated the witty observation by cyclists that the winner of the Tour is the cyclist who can eat the most! Cyclists searching for means to improve performance have used caffeine as it has been suggested that, in addition to its stimulant properties, caffeine may help modify metabolism to use fat as an energy source. However, objective studies have failed to demonstrate any benefit on any physiological parameters or total work time.

Stage racing

During a stage race any nutritional problems are magnified. Fluid replacement is extremely important because of the intense daily exercise and fluid depletion. Food intake is also difficult with the alteration of normal daily routine where it may be difficult to fit in three normal meals. Diet is therefore especially important during a stage race. Before setting out each day you should be well hydrated and passing clear urine. During the actual event you should be drinking, not just according to your thirst, but drinking greater than you would normally to avoid dehydration. Immediately after the race you should rehydrate immediately and throughout that evening should be sipping fluid.

While nutrition is important during a stage race, few of us race more than two or three major stage races in a year. It may be reasonable therefore during these stage races to ignore some of our principles of a normal balanced diet in favour of optimal calorie replacement. The most important aspect of the diet during a stage race should be to ensure adequate fuel replacement in the form of carbohydrate. It is difficult to eat enough natural complex carbohydrates to balance need as they tend to be bulky, so ideal fuel replacement has inevitable problems – such as trying to carry a plate of boiled potatoes with you. We may thus allow ourselves a little dispensation to eat some biscuits or sweets. After all, in spite of all the nutritional advice it is said that the most common nutritional supplement used during the Tour de France is gateaux!

After a race or training session, and particularly after a multi-stage event, the immediate post race period is critical for replacement of muscle glycogen. After a race the muscles are hungry for glycogen and in the one hour period immediately after an event the muscles are at their hungriest. You should aim to eat a snack as soon as possible after completion of the stage to ensure best fuel store recovery. There is no mystique or great expense in finding the most appropriate snack immediately after an event. The simplest snack and one which fulfils the principles of being nutritionally appropriate is sweet tea and jam sandwiches!

There are some rather unusual dietary rules handed down in cycling lore. One famous piece of advice is that you should not eat ice cream! This may have some substance in that ice cream has a relatively high fat content and perhaps some ice cream vendors may not maintain the highest hygiene standards. However most of us enjoy an occasional ice cream and there is no reason why we should not enjoy our sport and our food also.

The correct diet for a stage race should contain plenty of fluid, bread, potatoes, pasta, fruit and vegetables with a dispensation for some high calorie foods. There are no absolute dietary rules in spite of what nutrition specialists say and there can be great variation in a diet while maintaining the correct balance.

FLUID

Avoidance of dehydration, through fluid replacement, is a prerequisite for top class performance. It would be useful to have some means to gauge when a cyclist is well hydrated and in fact, nature provides a very convenient means of measuring hydration, that is, by observing the colour of urine! The darker the urine the more dehydrated the athlete. On the days before the event you should be passing normal quantities of clear urine. The professional cyclist may consume 12 to 16 bottles of fluid during a seven-hour stage.

Professionals have learned that proper hydration is essential for performance and this is shown through their fluid intake during the stage and reflected in their ability to provide a urine sample quickly for drug testing. Doctors involved in medical control report that professionals have a serious and sensible attitude to hydration. Their fluid intake is huge, and sufficient to balance their requirements. In effect this means that even when they are required to pass a urine sample for the drug test they are well hydrated and can easily pass a sample, unlike many amateurs who sometimes have difficulty even after a short race.

Fluid intake and maintenance of hydration is just as important during prolonged training as during racing. It is interesting to note the results of an experiment carried out at an Irish squad training camp. Cyclists were invited to weigh in before and after a training session and to document their fluid intake during the session. In one training session of 100 miles, non-racing, in February, in the rugged West of Ireland one rider lost 3.5 kilograms of fluid weight although he had consumed 2.2 litres. The total fluid loss was therefore 5.7 litres. Bearing in mind that this was during a six-hour training session in the winter, it gives an indication of the need for fluid replenishment. For simple replacement of fluid loss alone, water is the fluid of choice. During a longer race however we may try to maintain some calorie intake and the optimum calorie replacement is through fluid. Drinks consumed during a race may thus contain some calorie replacement ie glucose. However the greater the proportion of glucose in the fluid the slower it will be absorbed. Thus in terms of fluid replacement there is a fine line between best absorption and calorie replacement. The most important feature of nutrition during the stage should be to ensure adequate fluid replacement. We lose fluid through sweating on a hot day but we also lose fluid imperceptibly through our breath and evaporation in the wind.

Sports drinks

Fluid replacement is an essential component of nutrition for all endurance sports and cycling is no exception. In an effort to seek some performance advantage cyclists may be encouraged to buy proprietary sports drinks. Sports drinks are big business, with endurance athletes targeted by marketing hype. There are many drinks available, each with enthusiastic claims about their ability to make athletes run faster, jump higher, and keep going longer. However there are few secrets in sports drinks and no magic formula for sporting performance. Many drinks are marketed as special sports drinks and most have something to offer but you must be aware of what you are looking for in a drink: is it simply fluid replacement or do you require some energy supplement? Is it for training, racing or for recovery? Each occasion has different needs and priorities and there are circumstances when fluid replacement is the priority and other occasions when energy, calories or food value are more important. It depends on the event and environmental conditions.

Pre-race fluid

Before competing in any endurance event you must be adequately hydrated. For two to three days prior to the event you should drink freely. Water is the ideal fluid. No additives, glucose or electrolytes are required, just plain water.

During the event

During an endurance event such as a cycle race, triathlon or marathon the optimum fluid is determined both by the environmental conditions and the duration of the event. It is important to guard against dehydration. Exercise generates heat and one of the adaptive mechanisms of training is an improvement in the body's ability to disperse heat. If exercising intensely in warm weather conditions, in a long duration event, you will sweat profusely to help maintain body temperature. Trained athletes can work harder, generate more heat, and also sweat more and thus fluid loss through sweating is essential to prevent overheating or hyperthermia. In very warm conditions you may lose up to one litre per hour of sweat. Even a three percent fluid loss through dehydration can have a remarkable effect on athletic performance so it is essential to avoid excessive fluid loss. Professional cyclists are acutely aware of the need for fluid replacement and may take 10 to 15 water bottles during a five-hour race in warm weather.

There has been some interest in the need for electrolyte replacement and many companies use this as a marketing strategy. However sweat is more dilute than the fluid in the bloodstream (plasma) so sweating in effect concentrates the plasma. Electrolyte replacement is therefore not critical during the event itself.

The use of electrolyte replacement in sports drinks after racing and training may be of value but probably unnecessary in practice as a normal diet of fresh fruit and vegetables, in combination with the normal salt usage in cooking, will usually provide adequate post-exercise electrolyte replacement.

In a long duration endurance event such as a four- or five-hour cycle race you will require some additional calories. Glycogen is the body fuel and you will have glycogen stores to last for approximately two hours. During an endurance event, in an effort to avoid running out of fuel, you may need to take on some extra fuel as liquid calories. Sports drinks may offer calorie replacement, often in the form of a glucose solution but there may be a problem as the more concentrated the drink, the slower it is absorbed from the stomach. We already know that in an endurance event fluid replacement is essential, so high concentration glucose drinks may be counter-productive if they prevent fluid absorption. In warm weather where fluid replacement is especially important, glucose concentration should be kept low to maintain optimum fluid absorption – glucose concentration should probably not exceed five percent. In an attempt to optimise absorption, drinks are manufactured to be the same concentration as blood. This critical concentration is known as 'isotonic', and an isotonic glucose mixture will be five percent glucose ie five grams of glucose in a solution of 100 mls water.

An isotonic fluid is well absorbed from the stomach. Fluids more concentrated than body fluid are known as hypertonic and if you increase the concentration of glucose to perhaps 10% to increase calorie content then unfortunately this fluid is absorbed more slowly. Calorie replacement will mean a trade-off against fluid replacement. In addition, high glucose concentrations are often less palatable and as you will probably have already found that when competing, drinks often taste much sweeter than when used in normal circumstances. Palatability is clearly an important factor in maintenance of hydration. In order to avoid this absorption problem, yet increase the calorie content of drinks, manufacturers have used glucose polymers to provide greater quantities of glucose and yet remain isotonic. Glucose polymers are long chains of glucose which, because the glucose is linked together, are better absorbed. For optimum calorie and fluid replacement these are probably the most appropriate sports drink at present.

One word of advice! As the concentration of sports drinks is so critical, it is vitally important to make up the drink according to the manufacturer's instructions.

Fluid and training

It is important to be aware of fluid replacement not only during racing but also when training. We all aim to gain maximum benefit from training so should be just as careful of our nutritional and fluid needs during training as during racing. Dehydration occurs not only in hot weather but can also occur during a long training session even in the depth of winter so fluid replacement is equally important during a long winter training run. In addition, the cumulative effect of regular intense training sessions may lead to chronic dehydration. One may gauge hydration from day to day by daily weighing. During warm weather hard endurance training you should weigh yourself at the same time each day and note any weight deficit. A short term weight loss means dehydration and if you lose half a stone on a training session you can be sure that this weight loss was not fat but fluid. Loss of fat occurs more slowly and short term fluctuations in weight are due to fluid loss.

Post exercise

After an event, it is important to ensure adequate fluid replacement. Even with free fluid intake during an event it is difficult to maintain perfect fluid balance so afterwards you should drink freely. It is not quite so important that the drink be isotonic, as the speed of fluid absorption is not critical, so glucose concentration is not so important. Indeed, it may be of value to use a high calorie drink immediately post exercise because the body can most easily replace glycogen stores during the immediate post exercise phase. The cells are most hungry for glycogen, the key enzyme, glycogen synthesase, is at its highest and a high calorie drink is the ideal high energy fuel during the immediate post exercise period. Alcohol is not a suitable fluid for rehydration as it has a diuretic effect and will leave you even more dehydrated.

High calorie medical nutritional drinks are used by some athletes. These may be of some value in high energy expenditure sports where it is difficult to achieve appropriate calorie intake, but most athletes ingest sufficient calories in a high carbohydrate diet. High calorie drinks may be of value where you have to compete in heats and finals extended over a day and where it is not possible to consume normal meals.

There is no magic elixir, no drink with any extraordinary qualities or one formulation that is appropriate to all circumstances. For fluid replacement alone, water is superior to any proprietary drink. During a longer event an isotonic drink may be of more value such as a five percent glucose drink or a glucose polymer drink. After exercise a drink with a higher calorie content is allowed and this does not necessarily mean a sports drink but may include even the proprietary soft drinks such as Coke, 7-up etc.

ALCOHOL

Alcohol is a mild sedative which in moderation causes relaxation and bonhomie. Alcohol in moderation will not impair performance, but tolerance varies between individuals. An occasional drink is not a problem but clearly any excess will impair your racing and training performance. Alcohol is a mild diuretic which means that it encourages the kidneys to produce more urine. Thus it may increase dehydration especially if drinking to excess. Excess alcohol may also impair the ability of the liver to store glycogen. Glycogen storage is the main energy source for muscle, and decreased liver glycogen handicaps energy supply and hence performance in endurance sport. Because alcohol in moderation may aid relaxation it has thus become part of sporting culture. However, it seems foolish to invest so much valuable time into training and preparation for sport to throw it all away by drinking to excess.

If you have a hangover you will be generally unwell and unable to gain the benefits from a training load. With a hangover you will be dehydrated, with a dry mouth, thirst, and will have an increased heart rate response to exercise. Moderate exercise intensity will cause a greater physiological load and intense high level cycling in training or racing will not be possible.

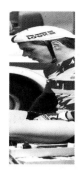

CHAPTER 13

DRUGS

There continues to be considerable publicity surrounding the use and abuse of drugs in sport. It is unfortunate that cycling has such a reputation for abuse of drugs that we must concede it is not without justification.

Paul Kimmage, the Irish ex professional cyclist revealed aspects of this abuse in his book *A Rough Ride* which was poorly received by the cycling hierarchy. Sadly much that was stated in his book was common knowledge: there was significant drug abuse in cycling. Some aficionados believed that this book damaged the sport by its revelations, or that the book may have been written for the wrong reasons. Whatever the reasons, perhaps we should listen to the author and appreciate that it must have taken great courage to write such a book and make an open confession about his own behaviour.

The Sports Council in the United Kingdom has supported the program of drug testing of athletes in many sports including cycling, producing educational material and conducting various lectures on the problems of drug abuse in sport. The Olympic Council of Ireland, conscious of the importance of the athlete's awareness of drugs has produced details of banned drugs, giving some examples of medications that could cause an athlete to inadvertently test positive.

If you are a competitor it is vital that you understand the classes of banned drugs and some problems arising from their inadvertent use:

STIMULANTS

These drugs are allied to amphetamines known as 'speed' and have a stimulant effect. They also have a psychological effect which leads the cyclist to have more aggression, less fatigue and an exaggerated perception of their own ability. They are addictive however and can have adverse side effects.

It is possible for a cyclist to test positive for a banned drug in this group without deliberate abuse. Many preparations, such as cold cures and nasal sprays, which may be bought over the counter in supermarkets and pharmacists contain ephedrine or an ephedrine-related compound. These compounds are banned drugs. A cyclist may have been prescribed or bought them without knowing, but this is not a valid excuse if you test positive. It is even more important to be careful when abroad as it may be difficult to communicate with the pharmacist or doctor or even to interpret the contents listed on the packet. To avoid inadvertently testing positive, be very wary of nasal sprays and cold cures.

NARCOTIC ANALGESICS

This group of drugs includes Diamorphine (Heroin) morphine and allied compounds. These are strong painkillers and have been abused in the past. Needless to say they are prohibited but are also highly addictive. No sensible cyclist would ever entertain the idea of using these drugs to improve performance. However, once again, it is possible to use banned products without intention. For example Paracodol contains codeine, and codeine is closely related to the narcotic analgesics in chemical formula so is also banned.

ANABOLIC STEROIDS

An athlete is most unlikely to have an inadvertent positive result due anabolic steroid use and if the test is positive the athlete is almost certainly guilty of abuse. There are very few medical conditions where anabolic steroids would be prescribed appropriately and certainly not in a fit young athlete. There have been many celebrated instances of anabolic steroid abuse. Ben Johnson, the Olympic 100m winner in 1988 was caught positive for use of an anabolic steroid and some notable cyclists have also tested positive. Anabolic steroids have been used by strength and power athletes in weight lifting, throwing sports and in sports where muscle bulk is important. Their use in endurance athletes is less well known, but they have been used for their ability to aid recovery in periods of intense training and racing where they enable the athlete to undertake greater training loads and hence improve performance.

BETA BLOCKERS

No cyclist will use beta blockers. They slow the heart rate and will greatly harm performance in endurance sport. They have been used mostly in sports that require calm concentration such as shooting, archery and snooker. Some middle aged cyclists who suffer from high blood pressure or heart disease may be prescribed beta blockers by their doctors. These veteran cyclists need not worry about 'dope control', but it would be useful for them to discuss with their doctor alternative appropriate medication for their condition. Beta blockers will not only slow heart rate but will inhibit the training effect of exercise on the heart and prevent some of the benefits of exercise.

DIURETICS

This group of drugs is used to stimulate the kidneys to produce urine. They should not be used in cycling as one of the main problems for cyclists, particularly in warm weather, is in maintaining hydration and diuretics cause relative dehydration. They are of course a banned drug. There is no appropriate use among cyclists and their only use is likely to be in an attempt to produce more dilute urine to confound the drug test. However, it is useful to note that current drug tests are so sensitive that even minute quantities of banned drugs are detectable. Diuretics may be abused in other sports in order to reduce weight, where weight category such as boxing, weight lifting and lightweight rowing is important. Female athletes may be tempted to use diuretics to reduce premenstrual fluid retention but this is inappropriate in a sport where hydration is important.

PEPTIDE HORMONES

This is a new group of drugs open to abuse, sometimes referred to as 'designer drugs'. They are synthetically produced hormones, identical to the natural body hormones that control growth, muscle bulk and red blood cell production. They include growth hormone and Erythropoetin (EPO). Erythropoetin stimulates our bone marrow to produce more red blood cells which aids the oxygen-carrying capacity of blood and enhances endurance performance. However if used without medical supervision this drug may over stimulate the bone marrow making blood excessively thick and causing severe medical problems including potential blood clotting, strokes, and heart attacks.

BLOOD DOPING

This is a method of supplementing the body's natural pool of red blood cells to improve oxygen carrying capacity. Approximately 800ml of blood is removed and the body automatically manufactures more blood to make up the deficit. The previously removed blood is then retransfused and in theory the athlete can now perform better as there is a greater capacity to transport oxygen. There are risks of infection, adverse reaction, and overload of the circulatory system.

LOCAL ANAESTHETIC AND STEROID INJECTIONS

Local anaesthetic injection can be used within limited medical guidelines. They may be injected into local painful areas but may not be injected into joints.

Local steroid injections are glucocorticoids which are very different to anabolic steroids. Glucocorticoid steroid injections are used to reduce chronic inflammation and may occasionally be used in treating local inflammation. These may be used under limited medical guidelines but must be notified to the officials.

OTHER MANIPULATIVE PROCEDURES

There are many stories of attempts to manipulate the drug testing procedures by the use of drugs, catheters, tubes and condoms. Probenecid is a drug used to inhibit the excretion of anabolic steroids in the urine. This drug is banned, not because it can improve athletic performance but because it masks the use of other banned drugs. All physical attempts to manipulate the drug test are banned. This is why during testing the athlete must strip almost completely and why the doctor must actually observe the urine being passed into the bottle. Cyclists have been caught with tubes, catheters and condoms filled with 'clean' urine.

Those of us involved with sport from top level right down to local third category events believe in the concept of fair and equal sport. It would be ideal if it could be proven that drugs were not of benefit to performance or that the abuse of drugs had such appalling side effects that true athletes would never consider using them. Unfortunately drugs do work and although there are side effects they are not immediately obvious nor do side effects appear to influence the athlete's decision. Efforts to control the abuse of drugs in sport thus depend greatly on our perception of fair play and the willingness of our official cycling bodies to crack down on drug abuse with rigorous testing and realistic penalties.

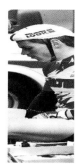

CHAPTER 14

AILMENTS AND MINOR HANDICAPS

Minor handicaps that prevent people from running and participating in other sports are not as great a problem in cycling. Because cycling is by nature atraumatic, with the body supported, it is an ideal sport to encourage participation by those who may have a minor handicap. Abnormalities and disabilities at the ankle causing immobility are not compatible with running but the bicycle, crank, pedal and shoes can be easily modified. Abnormalities in the gait or leg length differences may compensated by the pedals and shoeplates. Cycling is the ideal sport for those with joint disease as it allows exercise without constant jarring to the joints.

Spectacles

While in many other sports the wearing of spectacles is either too dangerous, inappropriate, or offends the macho image of the sportsman, wearing spectacles is very acceptable in cycling. Some of the famous world figures in cycling, including Laurent Fignon and Martin Earley wear glasses. Their reputation has changed the perception that those who wear glasses are wimps! And they may have even encouraged aspiring cyclists, proud to emulate their heroes.

If you wear glasses, because of significantly impaired eyesight, then you should continue to wear your glasses or contact lenses when cycling. You must be able to judge distances in traffic and your position in respect of other cyclists in the bunch. If you wear your own normal daytime glasses, you run the risk of these being broken by a flying stone or gravel, perhaps causing a more serious eye injury. Polycarbonate lenses are lighter, more expensive, but safer. They may be tailored to the same focal length as traditional spectacles. If you wear contact lenses you will know that there are two types: hard and soft lenses. Soft lenses may be worn for longer, are easier to put in and remove, and cause less problems for cyclists. They are unfortunately also more expensive.

Shades and sunglasses

It sometimes seems more important to 'look the part' than to be a skilful and powerful cyclist. 'Shades' or sunglasses are the trendy, almost essential cycling fashion accessory. They are expensive and flashy but they do have a very real and important function.

Eye protection is important. The eye is a sensitive and delicate organ and it is reasonable to protect your eyes from injury caused by grit, flies and the other flying debris on the roads. It is especially important in country areas where there may be cow dung or silage drainage on the road. A fragment of grit or an insect in the eye may temporarily blind you. This is irritating when training, but when racing may be dangerous if you wobble either into the path of an oncoming vehicle or upset the formation of the bunch. It is best not to rub the eye but to stop and if possible ask a companion to check if the offending grit can be seen. A companion may be able to remove the foreign body or wash the eye out very gently with pure clean water from a water bottle. Be careful and gentle. If the problem is not resolved seek help at a local casualty department. Sometimes the eye may have been scraped by a piece of road grit which may cause continuing pain or discomfort although the grit has been removed. Continuing pain should be investigated at hospital where the eye can be examined using a special dye and microscope. If simply due to a scrape of the surface of the eye, called a corneal abrasion, the treatment will be by eye drops and a pad.

If cycling in a sunny climate then it may be appropriate to wear eye protection. Professionals who spend six or seven hours per day cycling in bright sunshine, especially in the high mountains with glare, should protect their eyes from direct and reflected light. Ultraviolet protection will improve comfort even for any rider. Excessive exposure to ultraviolet light may cause a cataract. This is a cloudy deposit in the lens of the eye which may harm vision. A cataract is a permanent disability which may require surgery later in life.

Conjunctivitis

Conjunctivitis is inflammation of the white of the eye called the conjunctiva. It is usually caused by infection. You may wake in the morning with a sore, sticky eye and yellowish discharge and the eye may be slightly swollen and difficult to open. Most eye infections are viral but infection may be caused by contamination of the eye from road grit or insects. Antibiotic ointment or eye drops are the appropriate treatment. Most cyclists will find it uncomfortable to train or race when suffering from an eye infection as the wind causes pain and discomfort.

Hearing impairment

Unlike many team games where verbal communication is important, deafness is not an exclusion to cycling. During the race there is little opportunity or necessity for verbal communication, although those who are deaf should perhaps be accompanied during training, if only to warn of approaching traffic. In all cycling events the commissaire issues instructions through flags and there are always direction signs and visually displayed hazard warnings.

Ear infections

An acute ear infection causes a severe, often throbbing pain, in the ear. It may be associated with a respiratory infection or occur in isolation. Sometimes the eardrum may rupture and there is a smelly sticky discharge from the ear. Treatment is with antibiotics, occasionally with ear drops, and you should complete the entire course. Occasionally you may develop an infection in the outer canal of the ear which does not affect the eardrum. This is a common infection in swimmers known as 'swimmer's ear'. It may occur in any athlete however, especially if you attempt to clean the ear with match sticks, keys etc! An outer ear infection is treated with an antibiotic and anti-inflammatory drops.

Winter coughs and colds

Winter brings its share of coughs, colds, sore throats and ear infections. These relatively minor illnesses can interrupt your training and, if not managed correctly, can harm your fitness.

The most common illness affecting athletes in any outdoor sport is what we call the 'cold', or in strict medical terms an upper respiratory tract infection. Cyclists may refer to it as 'The Doom'! Symptoms may include a cough, runny nose, sore throat, sneezing and sometimes a buzz in the ears or reduced hearing. With a mild infection one may not feel ill but simply have mild symptoms and general discomfort. In the absence of a temperature, you may continue light training but it is important to balance the intensity and duration of training against how you feel. With a more severe infection, you may feel quite ill with, in addition to all of the above minor symptoms, quite severe muscular aches and pains. This indicates a more serious viral infection and the need to take greater notice of the illness. In these circumstances you should not train.

A golden rule that should be observed by participants in all sports is that you should not train when you have a raised temperature. If you have a temperature or fever this indicates that the body is attempting to fight the infection and you should rest, recuperate and allow the body every opportunity to recover. A mild infection without symptoms requires no treatment other than some pain relief and medication to keep the temperature down such as aspirin or paracetamol. With a more severe infection you should go to bed, with 'tender loving care' and plenty of hot drinks. The cold is a viral infection which means that antibiotics are of little benefit in treatment as a virus does not respond to antibiotic therapy. The best treatment of a viral infection is to ensure you have adequate rest which may enhance the body's ability to fight infection. One unfortunate fact about the cold is that there is not just one type of cold, but there are over 300 different viruses. Which means that having one cold does not give immunity to other cold viruses and it is quite possible to have one cold after the other. Sometimes an antibiotic may be necessary as bacteria may thrive in the mucus and secretions of the lungs, and may cause a chest infection. In this case you may cough dirty green spit, known as sputum. With a chest infection, an antibiotic is of value but requires a prescription from your doctor and you should complete the entire course.

If you have an illness that stops you training and you are frustrated by this inability to train you should remember that the aim of all training is improvement in fitness. We have already discussed the important training principle of overload and recovery. When you are unwell, not only are you unable to tolerate the load with no resultant improved fitness, but training when you are unwell may in fact harm your fitness level. When suffering from a mild infection you will not gain fitness by continuing light training: you can only hope to maintain some level of activity and general muscular tone and co-ordination. So, when suffering from a significant respiratory illness resist the temptation to clock up training miles and remember that you will gain nothing by trying to train, and by continuing to train you may even slow down your recovery and delay your return to quality racing and training.

Hay fever

Hay fever is an allergic condition that may affect the eyes and nose. The eyes feel gritty, water a lot and the nose may run with excessive clear fluid. Treatment may be by anti-allergic eye drops with or without antihistamine tablets. Both anti-allergic eye drops and antihistamines are permitted under drug testing regulations, but you must be very careful about using other preparations that may be prescribed or marketed for catarrh or nasal congestion. Many of these preparations contain substances prohibited under international doping regulations. Hay fever is common in cyclists, who are almost inevitably overexposed to pollen and other allergens in the countryside. Treatment is fairly simple and usually effective.

Sinus infections

If the skull were made of solid bone then it would be so heavy we would not be able to hold up our heads! In order to reduce weight while retaining rigidity, the skull is hollow in some parts. The cavities in the bone are covered by the same type of lining as is present on the inside of the nose, called mucus membrane. These bone cavities are known as sinuses and are connected to small tunnels which open out into the back of the nose. When you have a cold or respiratory infection the mucus membranes of the nose become swollen and block the openings of the sinuses. The mucus in the sinuses may become infected, inflamed, and the resultant swelling cause discomfort and pain. The symptoms may include a headache, usually at the forehead or behind the eyes, often throbbing, and usually worse on shaking the head. This is called sinusitis and it seems that cycling in winter, particularly during cold and wet weather, is more likely to cause irritation and inflammation of the nose lining, leading to sinusitis.

The treatment is twofold: treatment of the infection which requires antibiotics, and reduction of the swelling of the mucus membranes, perhaps with a nasal spray to reduce swelling. Be careful! Many of the medications available for the treatment of nasal congestion contain drugs that are banned under the regulations governing doping in sport. The older traditional treatment with inhalation of Friars Balsam or Menthol and Eucalyptus on hot water is just as effective and is permitted. Cyclists appear to suffer more frequently from sinus infections probably due to nasal mucosa hypertrophy.

Headaches

Some athletes suffer severe headaches following training or a hard race. There is a form of migraine known as 'post exercise migraine' which can occur after severe exertion. It may be treated with a mild painkiller. If 'post exercise migraine' is an ongoing problem it is possible to take prophylactic medication or drugs to prevent the headache occurring. Be sure to tell your doctor that you are an endurance athlete as some of the medications can harm athletic performance and your physiological response to exercise. Post exercise migraine is often worse in the cold weather and it may be useful to ensure that your head and forehead in particular are kept warm during training and racing by wearing a thermal balaclava or a broad sweat band under your helmet.

Diarrhoea and vomiting

This is usually a viral infection of the gastrointestinal tract which may last 24 to 48 hours. The most appropriate treatment for mild attacks is to reduce your food intake and more importantly to increase your fluid intake as there may be considerable fluid loss. This fluid loss may be replaced by drinking cooled boiled water or one of the proprietary fluid and electrolyte drinks such as Dioralyte, Rehidrat etc. The time tested classic fluid replacement is with flat cola and mixed water (50:50). Diarrhoea and vomiting may take two to three days to clear and will often disrupt training as you usually feel quite ill, both during the illness and for a few days afterwards. It is particularly important not to train in hot weather as the combination of fluid loss through illness and sweat may worsen dehydration.

Constipation

Most athletes in endurance sports are aware of the need to consume an appropriate diet and during normal training consume healthy foods high in natural fibres and cellulose. During a stage race or periods of intense training many cyclists tend to eat 'rubbish' foods, high in sugar with little fibre. This change in diet combined with relative dehydration may slow down bowel activity and cause constipation which may be in turn accompanied by crampy abdominal pain.

Constipation is best treated by increasing dietary fibre, through eating more roughage in the diet and improving hydration. The easiest method of increasing roughage in the diet is by eating more natural foods. Nature packs carbohydrate in fruit and vegetables with sufficient fibre to maintain normal bowel activity. Increasing the proportion of natural fruit and greens in the diet, supplemented by an increase in wheaten bread is usually sufficient. Bran may be added to or form an integral part of proprietary breakfast cereal.

The next step in managing constipation is by medication. Senna tabs or Senakot may be bought over the counter in a pharmacy and other medications are available from your doctor.

Haemorrhoids

Piles or haemorrhoids are painful itchy swellings at the edge of the anus or back passage. They may become swollen, tender, extremely itchy and bleed. They are a form of varicose vein at the anal margin. No one knows what causes them, although they appear to be more common in cyclists and those with sedentary occupations. For mild haemorrhoids causing itch various creams are available although the most effective are those which must be prescribed by your doctor. Some more basic medications may be purchased from a chemist. More severe piles may require hospital treatment through injection or by another treatment known as banding. These are outpatient treatments, but occasionally haemorrhoids require inpatient surgery.

A haemorrhoid may suddenly become swollen and acutely painful. This is known as a thrombosed external haemorrhoid and is caused by a sudden bleed into a pile. The pile looks and feels like a bulging black grape and is acutely tender and the patient cannot sit on a chair let alone a bike. This condition needs medical treatment, first with ice, but often by surgical release of the swelling which gives immediate ease by relieving the pressure in the haemorrhoid.

Severe recurrent piles causing ongoing problems may warrant surgical removal. The operation is rather uncomfortable and you will miss at least 2-3 weeks training and perhaps more. However, with intractable piles, surgery is often the best long term solution, seldom regretted.

Cold toes

Cold and numb toes may be due to compression by foot straps that are too tight across the top of the foot. If the toestrap is too tight then blood flow to the forefoot may be restricted and the foot feels cold and numb. This compression may be eased by relaxing the straps or changing the type of pedal from the clip and toestrap to the clipless type. Naturally it occurs mostly in the cold weather.

Very cold toes!

Sometimes in very cold weather the feet may become extremely cold, even frost-bitten. When cycling your feet are quite static and although there is increased blood flow to the leg muscles there may be poor circulation to the feet which become numb and very white with complete loss of feeling. Because of this numbness, care must be taken in warming your feet. If warming the feet in water, ensure that the temperature is not too hot, as the numbness and loss of sensation may cause you to scald your feet without knowing. Sensation gradually returns as your feet warm up and sometimes with the return of sensation there is an intense burning pain.

Frostbite

Sometimes in very cold weather the feet may become extremely cold even frostbitten. In cycling the feet remain quite static and although there is increased blood flow to the leg muscles there may be reduced circulation to the feet. The feet may become numb, with complete loss of feeling and turning very white. Because of the numbness care must be taken in warming the feet. If warming the feet in water, ensure that the temperature of the water is not too hot before immersion. One may easily scald the feet without knowing due to the numbness and loss of sensation. It is best to warm the feet slowly and gradually. The sensation in the feet will slowly return but sometimes as the feet warm up there is intense burning pain. Flesh and muscle are mostly made of water and frostbite means that the tissues in the flesh are frozen. The tissue freezes and as frozen water swells, the tissues can be damaged. Reheating should be gradual and if there is severe frostbite or any anxiety, medical help should be sought.

Sunburn

Most cyclists spend at least three hours training or racing every Saturday and Sunday throughout the season. More serious cyclists will spend considerably more time both training and racing and even in temperate climates this means exposure to sunlight through the middle of the day when ultraviolet light penetration is greatest. We are becoming more and more aware of the risk of excess sunlight and its association with various skin cancers. It is well known that certain forms of skin cancer are more common on the exposed areas of the body in people who work outdoors.

There have been reports of skin cancer occurring in cyclists not only on the face and hands which are the most common areas but also on the front of the thigh. Ultraviolet light penetration not only occurs on hot and sunny days but may also occur on relatively overcast days in the height of summer. It would be prudent for cyclists to use skin protection when exposed for frequent or for long periods in training or racing. Sun creams are graded according to their screening potential so that for example one may purchase a sunscreen with factor 10. The higher the skin protection factor the more effective the sunscreen. Sun screen is particularly important in those countries where there is relative reduction of the atmospheric ozone layer. It is not only advisable, but essential, to use very high protection factor sunscreen when competing in New Zealand. Cyclists should note that massage creams, oils, and 'rubs' usually do not offer sunscreen protection.

Heat stroke

Heat stroke is unusual in cyclists especially in this country. Racing speeds seldom drop below 20mph so there is constant heat loss by convection in the wind. There will be little heat loss by conduction or radiation but some heat loss by evaporation. The constant relative wind speed helps protect the rider from overheating. You will gain heat when working hard yet going slowly which is precisely what happens when going uphill. Because cycling clothing is, in general, designed to prevent heat loss the climber becomes very warm and begins to sweat excessively. Unfortunately when reaching the summit of the climb the reverse climatic conditions apply. The cyclist descends rapidly with great heat loss in the wind, but no heat generation as there is little muscle activity. Thus a cyclist who crossed the summit bathed in sweat may reach the bottom of the descent cold and shivery even on a moderately warm day. These circumstances are greatly magnified on the steep climbs of the major professional tours where extreme heat from strong sunlight combined with heat radiating from the road and mountain rocks in the still air can cause great distress. Riders douse themselves in water, not so much for the immediate cooling effect, but to aid temperature regulation through heat loss by evaporation.

At the summit it is traditional to stuff newspapers into rider's jerseys to give them some insulation on the descent. The heat loss is such that on some of the descents of the Giro d'Italia in severe weather, cyclists have been so cold and shivery they have had great difficulty steering their bikes.

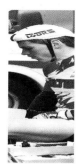

CHAPTER 15

YOUNG CYCLISTS

There are problems in determining appropriate age categories and distances for racing and training in underage cyclists. While efforts are made to encourage increasing numbers of younger cyclists to take up the sport there have been problems in overtraining and over racing which has seen a drop in the numbers of younger cyclists making their way through to senior ranks. There have been attempts in recent years to alter the rules of racing for underage riders. It is well recognised that there are risks to minors from excessive training and racing and the recent rule changes have been an attempt to protect them. Rule changes have not always been welcomed and indeed it may be that at times they have not achieved their objective. One of the reasons why a general rule does not fairly protect all is because of the great variation found in a particular age band.

Puberty can vary between the ages of 12 to 16 years so within each age group there may be wide variation in maturity irrespective of age. Some athletes mature early whereas others take some time to develop. Age group competition may sometimes be unfair as a more mature athlete will have better developed muscle strength, be bigger, stronger and win consistently. If a less mature rider competing within his age group is constantly beaten it may be difficult to maintain interest and enthusiasm for the sport. Yet, this athlete may have the potential to mature into a first class cyclist but be lost to the sport before developing their potential. Those who shine in age group racing may not be the champions of the future but simply early developers.

OVERUSE INJURIES

Before skeletal maturity, while bones are still growing, muscle is stronger than bone. Immature bones are relatively soft and constant high muscle tension can cause inflammation at the point of attachment of the muscle. This occurs simply due to muscle traction. It is called traction apophysitis and can occur at many sites in the body and is associated with various sports. In cyclists the major problem occurs at the knees where the quadriceps muscle on the front of the thigh is attached to the kneecap and the tendon in turn is attached to the top of the tibia, the larger bone of the lower leg. There is often a tender bony lump at this point in young cyclists. This condition is known as Osgood-Schlatters disease and is due to overuse. It will do little harm in the long term, but may stop the cyclist from training and racing. Overuse injuries are inevitable if the rider has been training intensively and racing at an early age.

HEAT LOSS

One of the most important psychological mechanisms that determines a young cyclists ability to cope with racing and training is temperature regulation; the ability to stay cool (literally). Younger athletes do not cope well with heat regulation so find it difficult to cope with high mileage and warm weather.

PSYCHOLOGICAL PROBLEMS

Children are always willing to do what is asked of them and if asked to race 60 miles will race without complaint. Often the main problems are due to the demands made by adults, parents, coaches and administrators. Children are naturally competitive but they are also sensitive. There may be a temptation for adults to relive their racing days through children thus putting too much pressure on them. A child may find the constant stress of racing, before psychological maturity, very difficult.

THE HEART

There has been concern at the risks to the heart by excessive racing and training. These risks may have been exaggerated. In view of their low body weight and relatively larger heart, younger athletes may in fact be better able to adapt to cardiovascular load than adults.

TRAINING AND RACING

The traditional cycling 'club run' may be a contributing factor to overtraining young athletes. Every young cyclist's first goal is to complete the club run with the seniors. To stay with the bunch, they must cycle relatively harder than older more experienced club mates; while the others are idling along, they may be at their limit just keeping up. When the bunch speeds up later in the run they may 'go out the back door' many miles from home, psychologically deflated and exhausted. Less intense or graded club runs of lesser mileage would be more appropriate. Grading racing is not the only problem, there should also be awareness of the problems in training and while it is impossible to lay down regulations for training, it is notable how few clubs have a policy for training underage riders.

Young cyclists are generally not well equipped physically and mentally to cope with intensive and extensive training or the frequent racing that older athletes perform. There should be guidelines to prevent racing too often and too hard, and to protect younger cyclists from the over enthusiasm of adults. On the other hand, if young riders do not race they may find they have no option but to go out on the club run with older cyclists going too far, too hard and for too long.

It seems reasonable to expect controls or restrictions on racing without restricting the enthusiasm of young riders. Our young riders of today are the racers of the future. It is better to enjoy the sport and develop than to become discouraged by too much racing, overtraining or injury.

Protect them from adults, however well meaning!

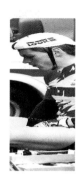

INDEX

a

abnormal tracking, knees,	26
abscess	59
Achilles tendinitis	34
acute panniculitis	
see saddle sores	
adductor stretch	56
aerobic capacity	46
aerobics	93
aerodynamics	45
alcohol	17, 105
allergies	115
anabolic steroids	107
anatomical snuffbox	22
ankle sprain	16
antibiotics	113
anti-inflammatories	31, 33, 35
antihistamines	82
anus	117
aspirin	82,
athletes foot	59

b

back stretch	56
backache	72
bench press	75
beta blockers	108
boils	59
bran	117

c

cadence pedalling	26, 49
calcaneous	34
calf stretch	55
calories	81
replacement in fluid	101
carbohydrate diet	81
chondromalacia patella	26
clavicle	see collar-bone
climbing	28
clothing, care of	61, 94
codeine	107
cold cures	107
cold feet	37
collar-bone fractures	23–25
compression treatment	15
concussion	17
conjunctivitis	88, 113
contact lenses	112
cramp	36
crankshafts	27
Criterium riders	66
cross-country skiing	92
cycling position	27, 37

d

dehydration	102, 104, 116
depression	70
designer drugs	108

Dioralyte	116
disc problems	40
diuretics	108
drinking to excess	105

e
Earley, Martin	111
ears	88, 113
elbows	22
electrolytic drinks	102–103
elevation, of injury	15
endurance riding	46
energy needs	66
equipment, maintenance	10
Erythropoetin	108
eyes	88
impairment	111
protection	112

f
Fartlek	65, 90
fast twitch muscles	51
feet	33
cold	37, 118
flat	36
femoral nerve	40
fibre, in diet	117
Fignon, Laurent	111
finger fractures	21
footwear	34, 59, 77
Friars Balsam	116
friction burns	13
fungal infections	60

g
gastrocnemious	34, 45, 55
gloves	see mitts
glucocorticoids	109
glucose drinks	103
gluteus maximus	44

glycogen	98, 103, 105
depletion	36, 67
replacement	82
groin infections	60

h
haemorrhoids	42, 117
hamstrings	44, 45
stretch	56
tendinitis	32
handlebars	19, 20
hard shell helmets	12, 58
headgear, types of	12–13
heart rates	49
estimating	63
heel tabs	35
hernias	43
Heroin	107
high pull	76
Hinault	53
humerus	22

i
ice application	15
injections, steroid	31, 35, 109
isotonic drinks	103

j
Johnson, Ben	107

k
Kelly, Sean	23, 25, 53
knee pain	25–29, 82

l
lactic acid	48, 63
leg length	111
LeMond, Greg	53
lifestyle	79, 96
loading in training	68

Lydiard, Arthur   62

m
marshals, motorcycle   11
menthol   116
migraine   116
mitts   21, 95
mountain biking   90
mucus membrane   115
muscle, balance   28
   blood supply   63
   fibre type   50–51
   spasms   36

n
nasal sprays   107
numbness, in fingers   19–20
   groin   42
NSAIDs   35

o
older cyclists   41, 58, 64, 108
Olympic Council, Ireland   106
orthotics   37
Osgood Schlatters   32, 122
overarousal   86
overload   64, 67
overshoes   95
overtraining   67, 69
   prevention   60
   treatment   71
oxygen uptake   47

p
palms, injuries to   20
paracetamol   82
paracodol   107
pedalling technique   33
pedals   27
   rotations   36

peptide hormones   108
Pes Planus   *see* flat feet
piles   *see* haemorrhoids
plantar flexion   45
position   37, 27
posture   44
   and wind drag   45
power clean   73
pressure points   19
priapism   42
probenecid   109
psychology   84
pulse monitor   64

q
quadriceps training   29
   stretch   56

r
radius   22
rectus femoris   45
rehabilitation   54
Rehidrat   116
respiratory infections   114
rest after injury   16
RICE in first aid   15
rowing   93
running   16, 54, 88

s
saddle height   45
saddle sores   41
scaphoid   22
scar tissue   21
sciatica   40
scientific testing   48
Senakot   117
sex   66
shoulder stretch   57
sinusitis   115

sit ups 75
skiing 92
skull cavities 115
slipped disc 40
slow twitch muscles 51
snacks, importance of 100
soleus 34, 45, 55
somatotype, elite riders 47
Sørensen, Rolf 23, 25
spine, flexibility 39
Sports Council 106
sprint training 66
sprinters 50
squats 74
squeeze pillow exercise 30
steroid injections 31, 35, 108
stress fractures 40
sun cream 119
surgery, knees 31
sweat rash 61
swimming 88

t
testing positive 106–107
thumb injuries 21
tibia 32
tibialis anterior tendinitis 36
toeing down 35
torsion of the testis 42
training load 26, 67
trauma to the hand 20
triathlon 91
turbo trainers 65

u
ulnar 22
ulnar nerve 19–20
ultraviolet 118
urine 101, 109

v
vastus medialis obliquus 28
VO2 max training 46–49

w
warm-down routine 54
warm-up routine 73
water 101
weekend training 78
winter training 78

y
young cyclists
  leg injury 32
  in training 68

Springfield Books is the UK's leading publisher of cycling and mountain bike books. The following is a list of the best titles in our current collection.

HOW TO BOOKS

Mountain bike racing, Gould and Burney, £10.95 (p/b)

Advanced mountain biking, Purdy, £14.95 (c)

Cyclist's body book, Westell & Martin, £12.95 (c)

Cyclo-cross, Burney, £12.95 (c)

Take up Cycling, Hendry, £2.95 (p/b)

MAINTENANCE & REPAIR BOOKS

Cycle Repair: Step by Step, Van der Plas, £8.95 (p/b)

Mountain bikes: maintenance & repair, Stevenson & Richards, £11.95 (p/b)

Bicycle Mechanics: in workshop & competition, Snowling, £11.95 (p/b)

GOOD READ BOOKS

Cycling Heroes: The Golden Years, Woodland, £17.95 (c)

The Great Tours, Watson, £19.95 (c)

Foreign Legion, Guinness, £16.95 (c)

Tony Doyle: six-day rider, Nicholson, £16.95 (c)

For further details regarding any of the above books or for a complete list of all our cycling titles, please contact

Springfield Books

Norman Road, Denby Dale, Huddersfield HD8 8TH

01484 864955   Fax 01484 865443